OPHTHALMOSCOPY, RETINOSCOPY and REFRACTION

BY

W. A. FISHER, M.D., F.A.C.S.
CHICAGO, ILL.
U. S. A.

Professor of Ophthalmology, Chicago Eye, Ear, Nose and Throat
College;
Late Professor, of Clinical Ophthalmology, University of Illinois;
Late Surgeon, Illinois Charitable Eye and Ear Infirmary;
Late President, Chicago Ophthalmological Society;
Member, Illinois State Medical Society;
Chicago Medical Society;
Chicago Ophthalmological Society;
American Medical Association;
Fellow, American College Surgeons;
Fellow of the Academy of Ophthalmology and Oto-Laryngology.

*With 248 illustrations including 48 colored
plates*

Published by
W. A. FISHER, M.D., F.A.C.S.,
31 North State Street,
CHICAGO, ILL.
U. S. A.

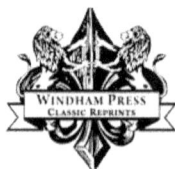

OPHTHALMOSCOPY,
RETINOSCOPY and
REFRACTION

INTRODUCTION

Ophthalmoscopy is generally considered as a difficult subject. It is one that is not taught either practically or successfully in medical colleges, with the result that scarcely two per cent of practitioners coming to the author for post-graduate teaching know how to use the ophthalmoscope.

In the author's opinion ophthalmoscopy and the fitting of glasses belong to the general practitioner, and acquirement of the necessary practical and theoretical knowledge is easy, interesting and within the reach of all.

This book has been written with the intention of teaching medical practitioners and students the practical use of the ophthalmoscope and retinoscope, with easy application of methods of study, to the detection of diseases of the interior of the eye, and for the fitting of glasses when they are indicated.

By mastering the methods here described and equipping himself with the necessary instruments, there is no reason why the general practitioner should not prescribe so as to correct the common errors of refraction and become proficient in the use of the ophthalmoscope.

The author desires to express his thanks to the staff of the Chicago Eye, Ear, Nose and Throat College, for valuable suggestions and especially to Dr. J. R. Hoffman and Dr. O. B. Nugent in the preparation of the chapter on Retinoscopy and to Dr. Carl Wagner on the fogging system.   W. A. F.

31 N. State St., Chicago.

CONTENTS

COLORED PLATES

N. B.—A duplicate set of Plates for use with the Schematic Eye is inserted.

OPHTHALMOSCOPY
RETINOSCOPY
and
REFRACTION

CHAPTER I

OPHTHALMOSCOPY

A complete examination of the eye cannot be made without a working knowledge of the ophthalmoscope; and diseases of the retina, choroid, and optic nerve cannot be understood unless the examiner is master of this inexpensive little instrument.

The author believes he has made the subject simple, interesting, and within easy reach of any physician or medical student. The student is urged to follow closely the method of instruction, since he will be expected to make a good ophthalmoscopic examination of his first patient.

If the student is expected to see the details of the fundi of the first patient examined, he must be taught the first principles of ophthalmoscopy on models. Medical men are usually deficient in their ophthalmoscopic studies and it is a hard task to instruct them upon living subjects. With the method now to be described, the student is taught the use of the ophthalmoscope in a surprisingly short time.

Ophthalmoscopy is usually taught to undergraduates upon the living subject in small classes; but it is difficult to get enough instructors, who can teach, to carry on the work successfully in this manner; and it is practically impossible to get the variety of cases necessary for instruction at any specified time even in very large clinics.

The author will place in the hands of his readers, a method of study whereby practically all diseases of the interior of the eye are observed in a model; and, when these have been mastered, the student will be as well prepared to examine the interior of any patient's eye and study the picture as he would that of any external disease, because they are just as easily recognized.

Medical men as a rule do not profess to know much about the use of the ophthalmoscope; and the majority of them believe it is practically impossible for them to learn its use within a reasonable time. This idea must be abandoned before any progress can be made.

Many medical men believe that lesions found in the interior of the eye which would come under their observation would be difficult to detect; but this also is not true. Many lesions found in diseases of the retina, choroid, and optic nerve are usually so pronounced in type that a diagnosis can be made on sight. It is the object of this chapter to show how they can easily be made visible.

Before beginning the subject of ophthalmoscopy, a description of the ophthalmoscope will be given; and, after that, the student will be

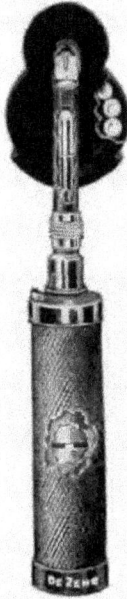

Fig. 1
Electrical Ophthalmoscope.

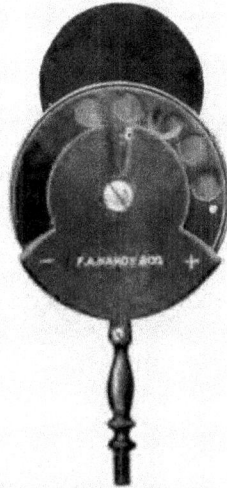

Fig. 2.
Loring Ophthalmoscope.

expected to understand the subject as he pro-
gresses, and not pass anything until he is master
of it.

THE OPHTHALMOSCOPE: In the diagnosis of
many diseases, including some conditions in the
domain of general medicine, which produce char-
acteristic changes in the interior of the eye, the
use of the ophthalmoscope, which is an instrument designed for the illumination of its transparent media and deeper structures making their
examination as simple and easy as that of the
external portion, is indispensable.

There are many models of the instrument, but any one which the doctor accustoms himself to is usually satisfactory.

ELECTRICAL OPHTHALMOSCOPE: It is easier for a beginner to illuminate the interior of the eye with an electrical ophthalmoscope, (Figure 1) which while expensive, offers some advantages.

The instrument most generally adopted in the United States of America is the Loring (Figure 2); and, in this work, it will be described and directions given for its use in the practice with the model.

LORING OPHTHALMOSCOPE: The essential parts of a Loring Ophthalmoscope are a perforated mirror for reflecting the light into the eye and two discs carrying convex (+) and concave (—) lenses.

The larger inner disc contains seven convex lenses, varying by differences of 1 dioptre (abbreviated D) from 1 to 7 dioptres, and eight concave ones varying similarly from 1 to 8 dioptres. Between the plus and minus 1 D. lenses in this disc is left an opening of corresponding size which contains no lens and is spoken of as the aperture. With these may be combined the lenses in the small outer disc which contains one each of + 0.50 D. and + 16 D., as well as — 0.50 D. and — 16 D. lenses. By combining the outer and inner discs, one is able to get any convex or concave lens from 0.50 to 24 D.

The unit of lens measure, the dioptre, mentioned above and frequently used throughout the text, has by international agreement been accepted as the strength of that lens which has its focus at a distance of one metre (40 inches). With the dioptric strength of a lens known, its focal length is ascertained by division into 100 centimeters or 40 inches, and conversely the dioptric measurement is arrived at by division of the focal distance into these same figures. Thus a lens of 2 D. has a focal length of 50 centimeters, or 20 inches; and one of 25 centimeters or 10 inch focal length is spoken of as a 4 D. lens either plus or minus, as the case may be.

The fundus of a normal eye can be seen through the aperture without any lens; but, if the eye examined is hypermetropic (far sighted), plus lenses are required; if myopic (near sighted) minus lenses are necessary to secure a correct view of it.

It is not necessary to have absolute darkness for ophthalmoscopy, but the darker the examining room, the better the illumination of the fundus and consequent ease of examination and accuracy of findings. In the sick room, drawing the shades will suffice; but in the office, the walls and ceilings may well be painted black.

DIRECT METHOD: To examine an eye with the ophthalmoscope by direct method, the examiner should be as near it as possible, keep both eyes open, and look into the distance with the examining eye through the aperature of the instrument. By doing so, he will learn to relax his own accommodation.

LIGHT: The interior of the eye must be illuminated and students find it difficult at first to

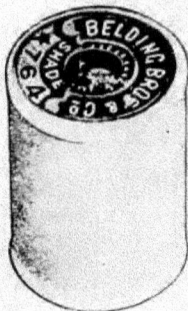

Fig. 3.   Spool

reflect and keep the light directed into the eye while making an examination. By practice, however, this can be learned upon the model as readily as one can by practice learn to shoot pigeons thrown from a trap.

ILLUMINATION: The simplest inexpensive method of mastering control of the illumination for the application of ophthalmoscopy is to practice reflecting the light from the ophthalmoscope into an ordinary spool (Figure 3) with the end toward the operator open and the other closed with white paper upon the inside of which have been placed black or red markings that can be identified by the student as he looks through the aperture of the instrument. After the student has learned to control the reflected light and is able to see through the perforation in the mirror, it is not difficult to illuminate the interior of the eye. The colored pictures that follow can be studied in the book and a working knowledge obtained, but a much better method is to study

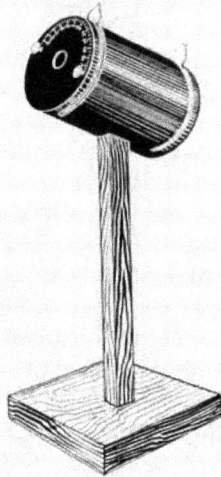

Fig. 4. Author's Practical Schematic Eye

the pictures in a special adopted model for the purpose.

A PRACTICAL SCHEMATIC EYE: (Fig. 4) can be made by any carpenter in the following manner. Select a piece of wood, round or square, $3\frac{1}{8}$ inches long and $2\frac{1}{4}$ inches in diameter; bore a hole $1\frac{3}{4}$ inches in diameter through it, and saw a slit through the barrel near one end to insert the picture, and another slit at the opposite end, large enough to insert a plus 13.00 D. lens from the opthalmoscopic case. The two slits should be two inches apart in order to approximate a normal eye. Two tacks, (one on either side) are driven into the front end with the heads projecting far enough to hold the lenses from the trial case, to be used for retinoscopy. Degrees

denoting the axis of the cylinder can be marked
on the model as they are made on any trial frame.
A stand can be made by making a base and an
upright and joining the base with the model, inserting one end in a hole made in the barrel, the
other in the base. The model can be painted as
desired, but the inside of the barrel should be
black; the stand should be made to give the model
an incline of about 30 degrees.

A picture is placed in the back of the barrel,
and in front a plus 13 dioptre glass from the
ophthalmoscopic case. In front of this lens is
pasted a piece of black paper or cardboard with
a 1.5 millimeter opening in the center to represent
the pupil. When proficiency is obtained with
the large pupil, another paper is pasted over the
first one with a 10 millimeter opening and when
the picture is easily seen, another paper can be
pasted over the last one with a 5 millimeter opening in the center of it. The pictures in the back of
the model can be studied with the ophthalmoscope, using any desired pupil until proficiency
is obtained.

To make ophthalmoscopy simple, easy, and
interesting, one should master the model before
looking at the eye of a patient. Retinoscopy
can be practiced upon the model with a 10 millimeter pupil, various strength lenses being placed
in front of the pupil. Duplicates of the 24 pictures are placed in the book to be cut out,
mounted on cardboard, with projecting thumb
piece for inserting; these are for use with the
model.

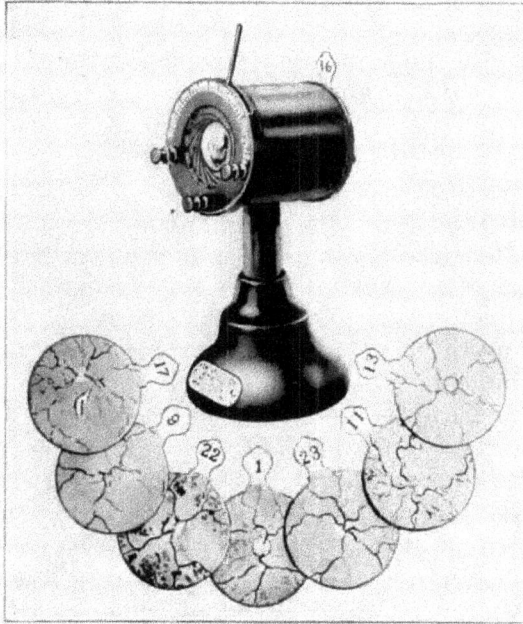

Fig. 5. Author's Schematic Eye.

The author's Schematic eye (Figure 5) is a model designed to make the study of ophthalmoscopy simple, easy and interesting. It consists of one cylindrical tube telescoping another one in such a manner that a long or short eye can be produced. If the two barrels are pushed together as far as possible we have a hypermetropic, short, or far sighted eye. If the two barrels are pulled apart as far as possible, we produce a myopic, long, or near sighted eye. If half way, —normal.

The model has a lens to represent the crystalline lens of the human eye, and an iris diaphragm. This iris diaphragm which when fully dilated produces a pupil of 30 millimeters, is made to open and close at the will of the operator and can be made to represent a normal, contracted, or dilated pupil. The beginner can commence his study with the maximum pupil and gradually decrease the size until it is much smaller than the pupil of a normal eye.

When the student has mastered control of the light and can examine the fundus of the schematic eye which is provided with twenty-four pictures, two normal and twenty-two abnormal ones, representing gross pathological lesions, he is ready to successfully examine the human eye.

EXAMINATION OF THE SCHEMATIC EYE: The direct examination of the schematic eye should be mastered before the student attempts the examination of a patient. If this be done and well done, he should be able to make a good ophthalmoscopic examination on the first patient seen.

To be a master of the schematic eye one should not only be able to distinctly see the fundus, but to know what to look for and recognize it when found as well. In the study of the individual pictures, the student should bear in mind that no great attention should be given to the color of the background of the eye, as this differs in a hundred cases, as one hundred faces differ.

The student should also understand that these twenty-four pictures were made to teach and impress the pathological lesions as well as the normal fundus on his mind. All of them were made to first represent normal fundi and are as different in color as three colors can make possible. After the twenty-four normal pictures were finished, twenty-two of them were made pathological but the normal part of the picture remains.

NERVE HEAD: The nerve head should be noted, but in actual practice much stress should not be placed upon its color. It frequently has a white scleral and black choroidal ring, which are normal and should be in the same plane as other parts of the fundus, not too high, "swollen nerve" or "choked disc" (Page 65) nor pushed back "cupped" as in glaucoma (Page 71).

NORMAL EYES: In normal eyes the vessels should emerge from the center of the nerve and not from the edge (Page 19). If they all emerge from the edge of the nerve, a picture of glaucoma is seen (Page 71). If some of the arteries emerge from the center of the nerve and some from the edge, there is a possibility of atrophy and the field should be taken.

THE RETINA: The retina is transparent and we need to observe its vessels only. The arteries are smaller than the veins, which accompany the former rather closely, the ratio of size being as two is to three. These vessels have no regular course and slight deviations should not be noted. By referring to the twenty-four pictures which follow, it will be seen that in no two are the retinal vessels the same.

WORKING PLAN: Before beginning the study

of the individual pictures a general working plan
of using the ophthalmoscope should be adopted.
The student must be able to determine whether
an eye is hypermetropic or myopic before he can
detect gross pathological lesions.

Working with the schematic eye, one should
measure refraction by the image of the screen—
the stippling seen in the picture. When colored
pictures are printed, a screen is used; and, when
we magnify these pictures with the ophthalmoscope, its image is easily seen. In fact one cannot help seeing it and this image is observed in
the measurement of the refraction instead of the
white lines on the arteries in the human eye.

TWO RULES TO REMEMBER

FIRST—HYPERMETROPIA: The strongest convex (+) lens with which the screen can be seen
at all represents the measure of the hypermetropic, "far sighted" "short eye" produced
when the barrels of the schematic eye are fully
closed.

SECOND—MYOPIA: In myopia "near sighted"
or "long eye" is produced when the barrels of
the model are separated beyond the point marked
normal (the more the separation the higher degree of myopia); the weakest minus (—) lens
with which the screen can be seen *at all* will be
the measure of the myopia, short sighted, or
long eye.

When the student can readily measure the
myopia or hypermetropia in the schematic eye,

set at any one of the numerous possible positions.
he will readily measure the refractive error in
the human eye.

POSITION OF THE EXAMINER AND THE MODEL:
The model should be placed on a table high
enough to be on a level with the examiner's
eye when sitting in an easy position, in front of
it. When using the right eye, sit in front of and
to the right side of the model and place the light
to its right side. When using the left eye, sit
in front of the model to the left and have the light
on the left side of the model. These are the positions one would assume if a patient was being
examined. (See Page 97.)

SOURCE OF LIGHT: The source of light may
be either an oil lamp, gas, or electric light with
a frosted globe, and should be on a level with the
model. The light should be placed upon a bracket that can be moved to either side of the model
as the student works with his right or left eye, and
which can be moved up or down in order to get
the desired light.

SIZE OF PUPIL IN THE SCHEMATIC EYE: The
pupil in the schematic eye can be made so wide
that anyone can see the picture in the back of
the model the first time it is examined; the
pupil can be reduced gradually as proficiency is
acquired.

DISTANCE FROM THE MODEL: When looking
into a room through a key-hole, the closer the
observer is to it the larger will be the field. The
same is true in looking into the model, or into

the eye; the closer the observer, the more he will see.

DIRECT EXAMINATION: With the room sufficiently darkened, the source of light and the model properly arranged, begin the examination by assuming the first position for direct ophthalmoscopy (Page 97), at a distance of about two feet; and, with the mirror of the ophthalmoscope tilted towards the source of light, reflect it into the pupil of the model, which at first should be made as large as possible; when the red reflex is seen through the aperture of the instrument gradually approach it coming as close as possible and assume the second position for direct ophthalmoscopy. The same position should be observed as when examining a patient. (See Page 97.)

WHAT TO FORGET: To make ophthalmoscopy simple and easy, the observer must first know what constitutes the normal eye. Forget the general color of the picture examined because the fundi of no two eyes are alike. They are as different as the faces seen on a crowded street; they all have eyes, ears, nose and mouth, but these all go together to make the face.

All fundi have a nerve head, and retinal vessels, but the color of the former varies so much that the observer should forget about its having a color as well as the color of the general background of the eye because of its variations.

Text books on ophthalmology usually devote so much space to describing the color of the background of the eye that the student soon becomes

confused. In this method, students are not expected to know or remember anything about the
color of the fundus.

THINGS TO REMEMBER: The student must be
able to measure the refraction of the eye before
he can make progress in diagnosis. The observer
always begins his direct ophthalmoscopic examination with the aperture, when he will be able
to see the screen in normal and hypermetropic
eyes.

SCREEN: If the observer can see the screen
with the aperture he will rotate convex (+)
lenses in front of it by turning the wheel on the
edge and will remember that the strongest convex
lens with which he can see the screen at all will
represent the amount of hypermetropia. If he
cannot see the screen with the aperture of the
ophthalmoscope he must turn on minus lenses to
make it visible; the weakest minus glass with
which he can see the screen represents the myopia.

RETINAL VESSELS: The student must remember that the retinal veins are one third larger
than the arteries and that the retinal vessels seem
to come out of the center of the optic nerve and
course across the fundus.

SCLERAL AND CHOROIDAL RINGS: There may
be a white scleral ring that the student can see
around the edge of the nerve and a black choroidal ring on the outside of it. These two rings
may vary or may not be visible and they sometimes appear to encircle the nerve head or only
part of it; but in no case are they pathological.

ATROPHIC AND PIGMENT SPOTS: If atrophic or pigmented areas can be seen that are nearer to the observer than the retinal arteries, these spots are situated in the retina. If the spots, either light or dark, are farther away from the observer than the retinal vessels; in other words, if the retinal vessels run over the spots, they are in the choroid. Remembering the things to be remembered and forgetting the things that are to be forgotten, the individual pictures will now be observed in the schematic eye; but before doing this, the student will be especially cautioned to remember two rules.

First, *the strongest plus lens with which he can see the screen in the model measures the hypermetropia.*

Second, *the weakest minus lens with which he can see the screen measures the myopia.*

It is very important to remember these two rules.

It will be natural for the observer to put on glasses with which he can see the screen best, but that would be wrong. The strongest convex (+) or weakest concave (—) lens with which he can see the screen *at all* is the correct one.

Ophthalmoscopy must be mastered before much progress can be made in the study of ophthalmology, and the student is urged to study the following pictures very carefully. They can be studied without a model but the use of this device simplifies the subject, develops skill, and makes ophthalmoscopy simple, easy, and interesting.

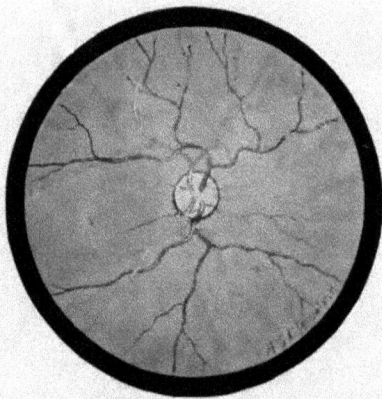

Dark Normal Fundus

PLATE I.

NORMAL DARK FUNDUS: Plate 1 represents
a dark normal fundus. The light streaks that
would be found in the human (retinal) arteries,
are absent as they are in all the following pictures. Otherwise it is a true reproduction of a
dark normal fundus.

RETINAL VESSELS: The retinal vessels are
seen emerging from the center of the optic nerve
and passing across the fundus in a normal manner, *the veins being one-third larger than the
arteries.*

THE NERVE HEAD: The nerve head appears
slightly hyperaemic but its color and also the
color of the whole fundus should be overlooked,
because it has been emphasized that the student
in his early studies should ignore the color of the
fundus and optic nerve.

When the mounted copy of the above plate
is studied in the model adjusted to make it either
normal or hypermetropic, "short" the screen will
be seen when it is observed through the aperture
of the ophthalmoscope. Plus (+) lenses should
be turned before the aperture of the ophthalmoscope as long as the screen can be seen and the
strongest one with which this can be done will
register the amount of hypermetropia. The
model can then be made long. "myopic" and the
weakest minus (—) lens with which he can see
the screen, will record the amount of myopia.

All of the following plates should be studied
in this manner in order to obtain practice in
measuring refraction because the eye must be refracted before any diagnosis can be made.

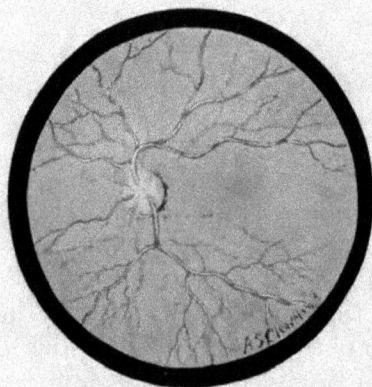

Light Normal Fundus

PLATE II.

NORMAL LIGHT FUNDUS: Plate II represents a normal light fundus with the retinal vessels emerging from the center of the optic nerve and coursing across the fundus in a normal manner.

NERVE HEAD: The nerve appears to have the same color as the fundus with a light spot in its center, the scleral ring extends half way around the nerve head on the nasal side, and the choroidal ring extends nearly half way around the nerve head on the temporal.

CHOROIDAL AND SCLERAL RINGS: The choroidal and scleral rings may be absent or much more marked in normal eyes, but they should also be ignored when looking for pathological lesions.

NORMAL FINDINGS: In this picture as well as Plate I, the student's attention is called to normal findings. The general background may vary from the lightest to the darkest and yet the eye remain normal.

This picture should be studied in the model in the manner described in the discussion of Plate I.

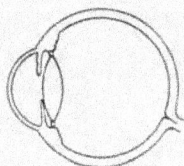

Fig. 6. Normal cross section

NORMAL CROSS SECTION: Figure 6 represents a cross section of Plate II. The student will notice that there are no elevations or excavations at the nerve head, or in any part of the fundus.

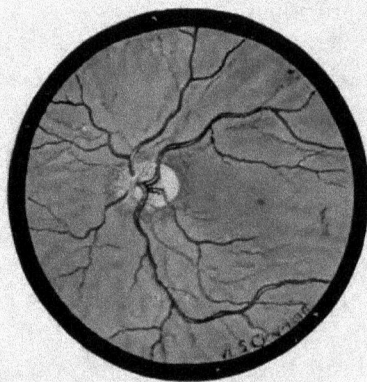

Myopic Crescent

PLATE III.

MYOPIC CRESCENT: Plate III. The retinal vessels are normal and the choroidal vessels, broader than those of the retina, show through the latter and there is a large white crescent on the temporal side of the nerve head. When such a picture is found in a myopic or long eye, a diagnosis of myopic crescent is made. Save for the large crescent at the side of the optic nerve, the picture is normal. In low degrees of myopia, the fundus often presents a normal appearance; but the above is very frequently found in high degrees.

DISEASES OF MYOPIA: The student is reminded that a variety of lesions may be found in high degrees of myopia, (near sighted eyes) such as choroiditis, uveitis, detachment of the retina, dislocated lens, and even general destruction of the eye ball.

CHAPTER II

DISEASES OF THE RETINA: The five colored plates that follow represent the commoner diseases of the retina, and they should be carefully studied with the ophthalmoscope in the model. The model should be made short, "hypermetropic" and the refraction carefully measured, then long, "myopic" and the refraction again measured. This should be done in order to acquire an idea of elevations and excavations, which must be done in order that a diagnosis can be made. This exercise will be found to be quite satisfactory upon the model.

It is the intention of the author to give the student and practitioner a working knowledge of ophthalmoscopy and describe a few pictures of lesions usually found in the fundus; the rare ones are not mentioned.

If the following pictures are carefully studied in conjunction with the use of the model, the student will be well prepared to make diagnosis of diseases of the fundus as he will meet them.

A beginner in the study of diseases of the eye is usually early in forming ideas regarding diseases of the fundus; he begins as a rule by imagining diseases that are next to impossible. If the normal eye and gross lesions are well understood, the lesser lesions soon become simple. A greater number of diseases of the retina would only have a tendency to complicate the subject.

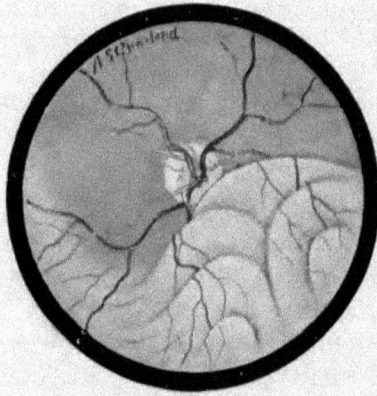

Detachment of Retina

PLATE IV.

DETACHMENT OF THE RETINA: Plate IV. There is a large white crescent extending more than half around the nerve head (Posterior staphyloma). The upper part of the fundus is red and the lower part is of a lighter color and is in folds.

The upper part appears red because of the choroid immediately under the retina while the lower part is of a lighter color, because the choroid cannot be seen, as the result of there being something between it and the retina. The retinal vessels pass over the entire fundus but the student will notice that they seem to be broken at the edge of the detachment, or at the junction of the light and red areas. A similar picture is seen in sarcoma of the choroid, but a striking difference is seen when comparing the retinal vessels of detachment with those of sarcoma. (See Plate X.)

A break will be observed at each fold of the retina in detachment, while in a sarcoma, breaks will be seen only at the junction of the light and red areas because of the absence of folds in the latter.

TENSION: In detachment of the retina the eye is usually below normal.

HYPERMETROPIA: In both detachment of the retina and sarcoma, the affected areas are more hypermetropic than the normal part of the fundus. If unable to make a differential diagnosis between the two conditions by the appearance of the involved retinal vessels, the doubt can usually be easily cleared up by puncture of the sclera

over the affected portion after cocainizing the eye.
If the lesion proves to be a detachment, fluid will
escape and the retina will be temporarily replaced
in position as can be determined with the ophthalmoscope. Should it be sarcoma, there will be no
change in position or size of the tumor.

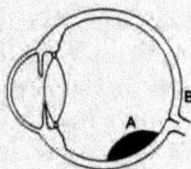

Fig. 7.   Detachment of Retina.   Cross section Plate IV

Figure 7 represents a cross section of Plate
IV. The student will note the elevation or hypermetropia of the detached portion. If the refraction is made with the ophthalmoscope at (A)
and then at (B) without removing the ophthalmoscope from the eye, the difference in the refraction will be easily measured.

ELEVATION: When measuring the refraction
of two portions of the fundus, a refractive difference of 3 D. is equivalent to a difference of 1
millimeter in level. The student will shortly
become adept at estimating the height of any
elevations or depth of any depressions he may
meet.

PROGNOSIS: Usually blindness.

TREATMENT: Rest in bed, laxative, sweats,
potassium iodide, sub-conjunctival injections of 1
to 3% salt solution or 5% citrate of soda; draw

off fluid by puncture or trephine the sclera after laying back the conjunctiva and exposing it, after which the opening is closed with one or two sutures.

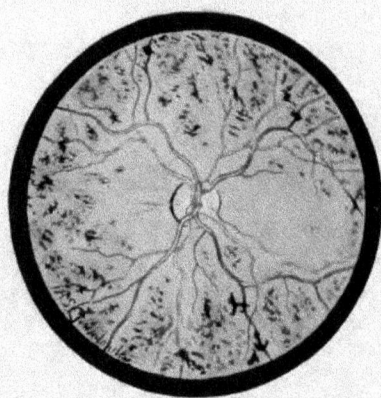

Retinitis Pigmentosa

PLATE V.

RETINITIS PIGMENTOSA: Plate V. The retinal vessels are normal and the scleral and choroidal rings are plainly visible. The background of the fundus is dark, spots of pigment are noticed, which are seen to be deposited on the retinal vessels. When the fundus is examined with the ophthalmoscope, the retinal vessels disappear first, when plus glasses are used, showing clearly that the spots are in the retina.

There is no difference in the ophthalmoscopic pictures of retinitis pigmentosa and acquired syphilis: but the former always appears in childhood showing itself symptomatically by complaint of the early onset of darkness toward the close of the day, even long before normal individuals note any failure of the illumination. This symptom alone occurring in a child is sufficient for a positive diagnosis of retinitis pigmentosa without the ophthalmoscopic picture. External examination does not reveal any symptom of disease.

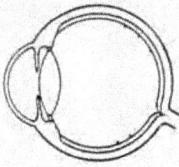

Fig. 8
Retinitis Pigmentosa. Cross Section Plate V.

Figure 8 represents a cross section of Plate V. The student will note that the pigmented spots are in front of the retinal vessels and can easily be distinguished from choridal pigment by measurement of the refraction of one or more of the spots and of an adjacent normal area with the ophthalmoscope as described on Plate IV.

PROGNOSIS: Blindness usually occurs about middle life or a little later.

TREATMENT: No treatment has as yet been found to be of benefit. However, errors of refraction should be corrected.

RETINITIS PIGMENTOSA WITH OBLONG DISC
(Luetic Retinitis): Plate VI. This picture is
produced in acquired syphilis; occurring only in
adults and closely resembles retinitis pigmentosa.

The spots of pigment are plainly in front of
the retinal vessels; whereas, if they were in the
choroid, the vessels would be anterior to the spots.

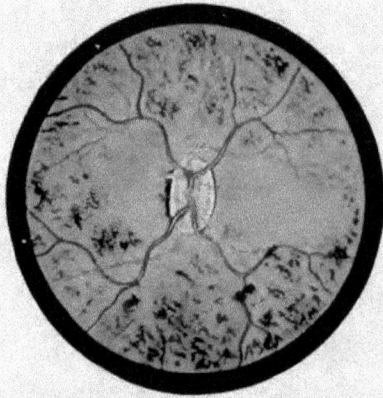

Retinitis Pigmentosa with Oblong Disc.

PLATE VI.

In observing the pictures in the model, the spots
will be seen after the arteries have disappeared
when plus lenses are introduced into the aperture of the ophthalmoscope, thus showing the
spots to be on the retina. The nerve head is
oblong to represent astigmatism, but it does not
have any relation to lues.

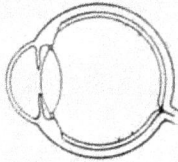

Fig. 9. Luetic Retinitis. Cross section Plate VI.

Figure 9 represents a cross section of Plate VI and is inserted to impress upon the student's mind the location of the pigmented spots. The student will recognize that it is not a difficult matter to determine their location with the ophthalmoscope. it being noted whether the spots or the vessels disappear last when plus lenses are introduced into the ophthalmoscope. If the spots are seen after the vessels have disappeared while increasing the plus, they must be in the retina; and, if the spots disappear first they must be in the choroid.

PROGNOSIS: If active but without too much destruction in the back of the eye, the process can often be arrested. If the lesion is old, the same treatment should be tried, but with less hope of improvement.

TREATMENT: If in a state of active inflammation. salvarsan or mercury and large doses of potassium iodide should be given; but if inactive. treatment of any kind is usually unsatisfactory. Errors of refraction if any, should, of course, be corrected.

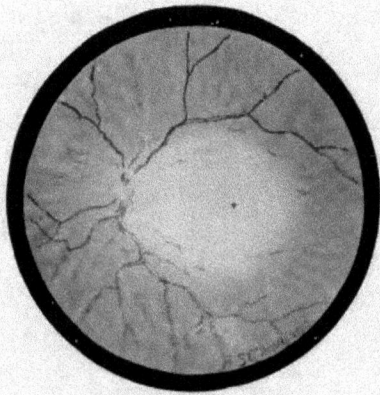

Embolism Central Retinal Artery

PLATE VII.

EMBOLISM OF THE CENTRAL ARTERY OF THE RETINA: Plate VII. The nerve head is blurred and there is a light area on its temporal side, covering the entire macular region, save for one small red spot. The patient gives a history of sudden loss of vision.

Figure 10 represents a cross section of Plate VII. The student will note that there is no

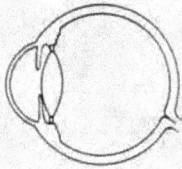

Fig. 10. Embolism Central Retinal Artery. Cross section Plate VII.

elevation of the fundus shown in the light area, as there would be if a tumor, exudate, or detachment of the retina were present. (See Plate IV and Figure 7.)

PROGNOSIS: Blindness in the affected eye without any external manifestations.

TREATMENT: Massage, paracentesis and iodide of potassium have been recommended; but the results are usually unsatisfactory.

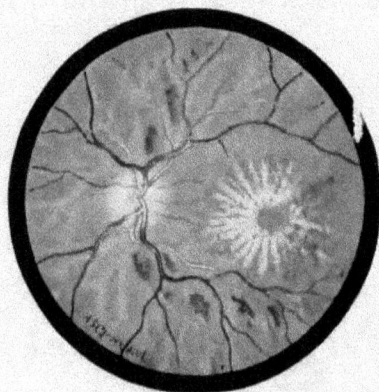

Retinitis Albuminurica

PLATE VIII.

DISEASES OF THE RETINA

RETINITIS ALBUMINURICA: Plate VIII. The nerve head is not swollen as in choked disc, Plate XX, XXI and XXII, nor is it pushed back as in glaucoma Plate XXIII and XXIV, but is pale as in atrophy Plate XVIII. The choridal vessels which are wider than those of the retina, can be seen through the latter and there are hemorrhagic spots scattered throughout the fundus.

The principal lesion, which is described as a stellate picture commencing in the macular region, is typical of this disease, is well marked and a diagnosis can easily be made by anyone who can reflect the light into the eye and illuminate its interior.

While this picture is particularly typical, most of the pictures of albuminuric retinitis are not so much so. The student should examine the urine of any patient in whom the diagnosis is not plain. Many diagnoses are thus made perfectly clear where only a slight lesion is found in the macular region.

PROGNOSIS: Very grave.

TREATMENT: General treatment of nephritis but with no hope of restoring vision. The urine, tonsils, teeth, sinuses and a general examination should be made for the source of infection.

CHAPTER III

DISEASES OF THE CHOROID: The eight following pictures fairly represent the disease of the choroid. They should be carefully observed in the model and the refraction measured in order to be able to make the all important differentiation between excavations and elevations.

If these eight pictures are carefully studied as described, very little trouble will be found in diagnosing diseases of the choroid when an examination of the patient is made; the author believes that more illustrations would only complicate the subject as designed for students and general practitioners of medicine.

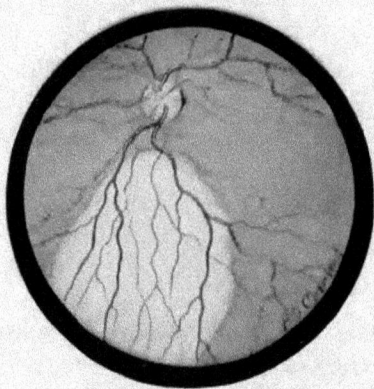

Coloboma of the Choroid

PLATE IX.

COLOBOMA OF THE CHOROID: Plate IX. The
scleral and choroidal rings are well marked. The
whole fundus is a normal red save in the lower
part which is white. The strongest plus glass
with which the screen can be seen on the red part
of the fundus would indicate the refraction at
that part of it, and the same measurement of its
white portion would indicate the refraction at
that point. If the red or normal part of the
fundus measured the same as the white it could
only be a coloboma of the choroid.

In this picture, the choroid is congenitally absent and the sclera is seen shining through the
transparent retina and the retinal vessels are seen
with a white sclera as a background. A coloboma
of the iris is often found with a coloboma of the
choroid, and presents the picture of a more or
less complete iridectomy.

The student is reminded to measure the refraction on the red part of the fundus which is designated as normal and without removing his eye
from the picture, to measure that of the white
part of the fundus.

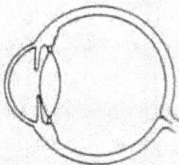

Fig. 11. Coloboma of
the Choroid. Cross
section Plate IX.

Figure 11 represents a cross
section of Plate IX. The student will contrast this picture
with figure 7 and Plates IV
and X. Here there is no elevation above the normal, while
in figures 5, 7 and 12 the elevation is well marked.

SARCOMA OF THE CHOROID: Plate X. The scleral and choroidal rings are well marked, extending all around the nerve head, the upper part of the fundus is red and the lower part light. The retinal arteries are seen to course over the red part of the fundus where the choroid is giving the fundus its red color as well as over the light part below, where there is something between the retina and the choroid.

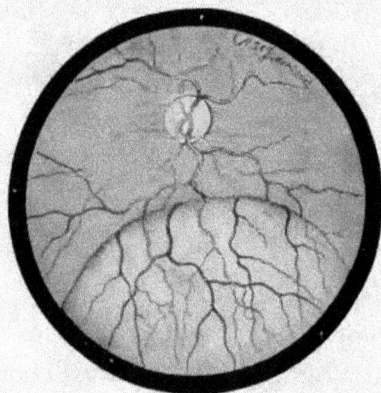

Sarcoma of Choroid

PLATE X.

HYPERMETROPIA: The sarcoma is always more hypermetropic than the red or normal part of the fundus. Compare with coloboma of the choroid (Plate IX), where there is a large light area in the fundus but which is not more hypermetropic than the normal.

VESSELS IN SARCOMA: There is a distinct break in the retinal vessels at the junction of the red and light areas such as is found in detachment of the retina (Plate IV). After the vessels have passed on to the sarcoma, there are no breaks as are found in the former.

TENSION IN SARCOMA: A sarcoma is not caused by low tension or soft eye as in detachment of the retina as it simply grows into a readily displaced watery body. The tension of the affected eye may either be normal or plus in the first stages of the disease. A sarcoma may become quite large without producing increase of tension, but later it always causes plus tension.

It is impossible to make a diagnosis of sarcoma of the choroid, without the ophthalmoscope, because the eye does not show any symptoms externally. If the vitreous and lens are clear the diagnosis is plain, especially with the use of the technique described for differential diagnosis under Detachment of the Retina (Plate IV).

Figure 12 is a cross section of Plate X showing the elevation of the sarcoma above the normal fundus. A, the elevation; B, the normal.

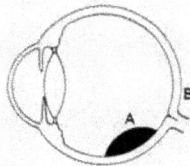

Fig. 12. Sarcoma of the Choroid. Cross section Plate X.

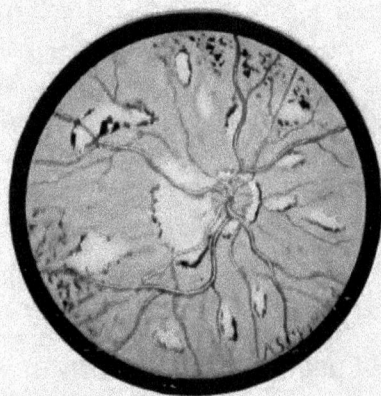

Posterior Staphyloma with Choroiditis

PLATE XI.

PROGNOSIS: The growth may recur in the eye socket after enucleation, or in some other organ.

TREATMENT: The eye should be removed and with it as much of the optic nerve as possible, followed by X-Ray treatment. If the tissues around the eye are involved, all the structures of the orbit should be removed.

POSTERIOR STAPHYLOMA WITH CHOROIDITIS: Plate XI. The retinal vessels are normal, the scleral ring is very large, and the choroidal ring is well marked. There is a large light atrophic spot at the temporal side of the nerve head, (posterior staphyloma); many white spots are scattered over the fundus, and the retinal vessels seem to run over them.

The spots are all choroidal; and, if the patient is myopic, the retinal vessels could be seen only with a minus glass. The student is reminded that in Plates V and VI the pigmented spots were in front of the retinal vessels while in this picture the vessels are in front of the spots. In those plates the lesions were in the retina; but in this picture the lesion is in the choroid.

PROGNOSIS: Rarely good.

TREATMENT: Glasses should be prescribed if necessary, but local treatment of the eye is useless. The urine should be examined and any general treatment that is indicated should always be given, having in mind the effects of lues upon the eye.

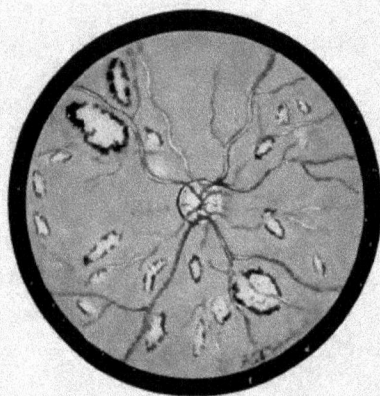

Disseminated Choroiditis

PLATE XII.

DISSEMINATED CHOROIDITIS: Plate XII. The scleral and choroidal rings are well marked and the nerve head is not swollen as in choked disc, (Plates XX and XXI), nor cupped as in glaucoma, (Plates XXIII and XXIV). The retinal vessels are normal. The only pathological lesions present are the atrophic spots in the choroid.

The sclera can be seen shining through the red choroid and the retinal vessels run over the atrophic spots.

VISION: The reduction of vision depends upon the location of the lesion in the choroid and the refraction of the eye. As long as the macular region remains free from disease central vision may be expected to be retained.

PROGNOSIS: Grave if macula is involved.

TREATMENT: Constitutional treatment and correction of errors of refraction.

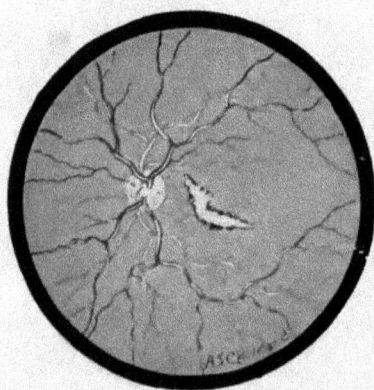

Rupture of Choroid

PLATE XIII.

RUPTURE OF CHOROID: Plate XIII. The retinal vessels and the nerve head are normal. There is an atrophic spot with a pigmented border at the temporal side of the fundus.

A diagnosis of rupture of the choroid, impossible at the time of injury because of hemorrhage into the vitreous, is made later from the ophthalmoscopic picture together with the history of injury.

VISION: Loss of vision depends upon the extent of the injury, and the location of the rupture. If it be on the temporal side, the loss of central vision will naturally be greater than would occur if the rupture were in some other part of the fundus.

PROGNOSIS: Depends upon the location of the rupture; the nearer the macula the less favorable the prognosis.

TREATMENT: At the time of injury two drops of 1% solution of atropin sulphate should be dropped into the eye three times a day together with such other treatment as is indicated. Potassium iodide is indicated for absorption.

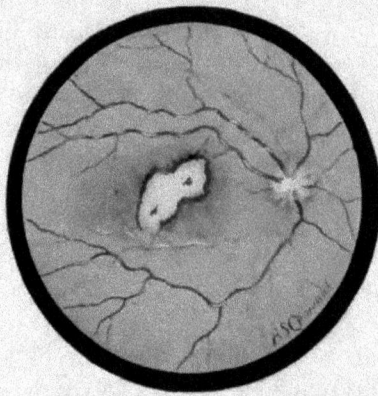

Central Choroiditis

PLATE XIV.

CENTRAL CHOROIDITIS: Plate XIV. The lesion represented here is an extensive choroiditis. It occupies the entire macular region, and it would be impossible for anyone to make a mistake in diagnosis, providing he had a working knowledge of the ophthalmoscope.

Such a lesion could be the result of trauma or any disease that would produce a choroiditis.

PROGNOSIS: Bad as regards vision.

TREATMENT: None.

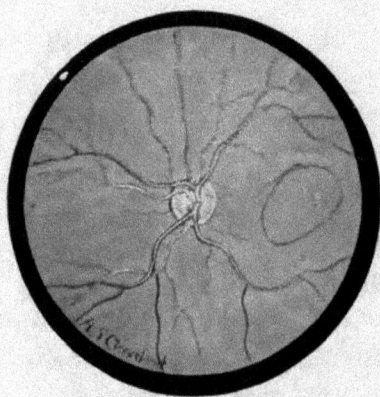

Central Choroiditis (slight)

PLATE XV.

CENTRAL CHOROIDITIS: Plate XV. The scleral and choroidal rings are well marked and the retinal vessels and nerve head are normal. Three small white spots are seen on the temporal side of the fundus in the macular region. A diagnosis of central choroiditis can be made because spots in this region, either pigmented or atrophic, are always the result of central choroiditis.

The fovea centralis is often very well marked but it is single and could not be mistaken for central choroiditis.

VISION: If the vision is normal there could not be a central choroiditis; but if the vision is reduced, a slight change in the macular region may be the cause of it.

PROGNOSIS: The loss of vision is usually permanent unless a specific cause is found and treated.

TREATMENT: Entirely constitutional.

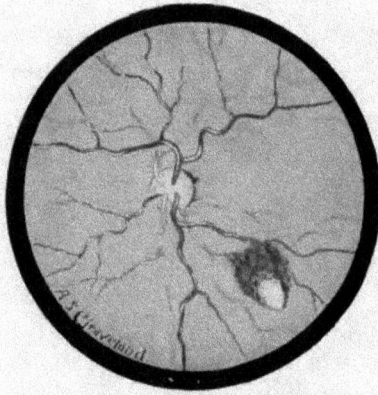

Injury

PLATE XVI.

INJURY—Plate XVI. This picture is that of a perfectly normal fundus, save that a piece of steel has penetrated the eye, becoming embedded in the sclera and is surrounded by blood.

A lesion in this location is not ordinarily as grave as if it were nearer the macula and produced by disease (Plates XIV and XV) : but in this case, the prognosis is very grave because of the lesion having been produced by a foreign body, which has been retained within the eye ball.

PROGNOSIS: Grave.

TREATMENT: Remove the steel with the giant magnet if the injury is recent and treat as any injury of the eyeball; sulphate of atropin 1%. 2 drops in the eye three times a day. If injury is of long standing enucleate the eye. X-Ray examination should be first made in all cases and foreign body localized.

It is not the purpose of the author to describe the treatment of injuries of the eyes; but it is always good practice to remove eyes that are blind and irritated, because the danger to the fellow eye is all important.

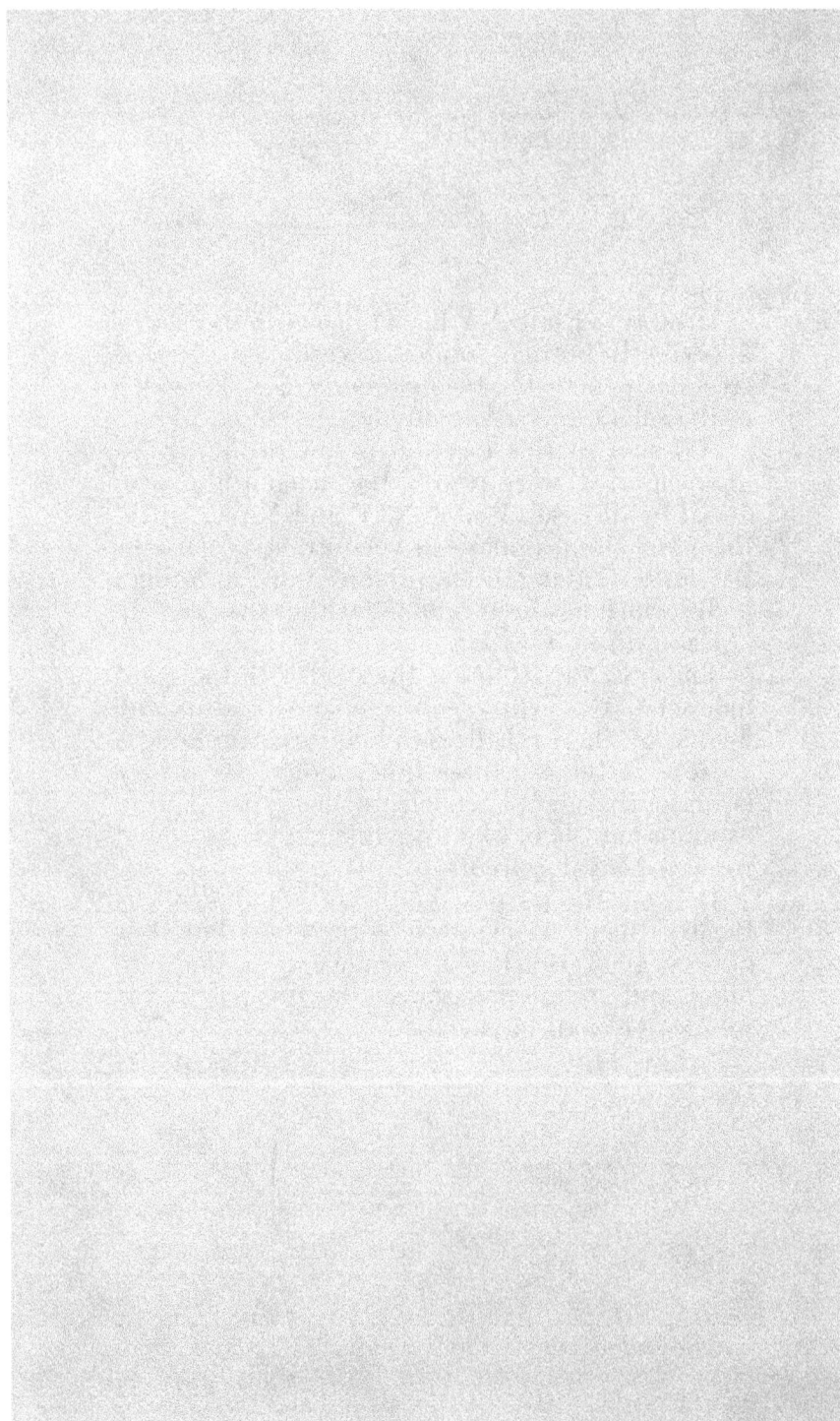

CHAPTER IV

DISEASES OF THE OPTIC NERVE: The following six colored plates with a consideration of the field of vision will give the student or practitioner a good practical working knowledge of diseases of the optic nerve. Diseases of the optic nerve can often be diagnosed only by study of the field of vision in conjunction with ophthalmoscopy.

More pictures than are here described would have a tendency to confuse the student and complicate the subject.

A discussion of the method of taking a field will be given on page 76.

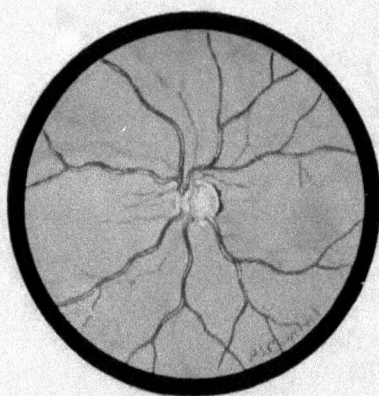

Glaucoma with Atrophy

PLATE XVII.

ATROPHY OF THE OPTIC NERVE WITH GLAU-
COMA: Plate XVII. The scleral and choroidal
rings are well marked but there is a marked
difference in the size of the retinal vessels. While
the veins are normal, the arteries are noted to
be small and threadlike. This condition alone
would justify a diagnosis of optic atrophy; but,
in order to be absolutely certain, the field should
be taken in each eye if enough vision remains to
make it possible.

This plate also presents a picture of glaucoma,
which condition will be taken up in a separate
chapter, the cupping of the nerve head being
shown by the apparent dipping down of the
retinal vessels at its margins and proved positively by measurement of the refraction as described under detachment of the retina. (Plate
IV.)

PROGNOSIS: Of optic atrophy grave. Glaucoma, see page 71.

TREATMENT: Atrophy-Salvarsan or mercury
and large doses of potassium iodide may be tried;
but, if a positive diagnosis of atrophy has been
made, treatment is usually useless. Strychnia is
recommended by some.

If glaucoma, see page 71.

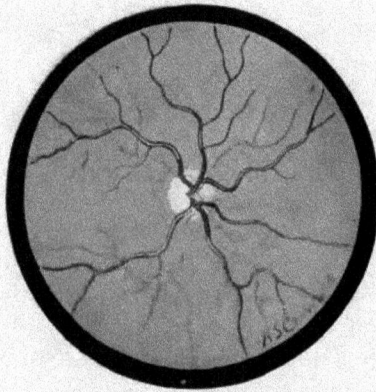

Optic Atrophy

PLATE XVIII.

OPTIC ATROPHY: Plate XVIII. The student
has been cautioned regarding the color of the
optic nerve in atrophy; but, in this picture the
patient is blind which prevents taking the field
and the diagnosis must be made from the white
disc and threadlike arteries. The veins are normal in size.

FIELD: If the patient can see well enough to
permit the taking of the field, it should always
be done in each eye. When a concentrically
contracted field is found the student can be sure
of his diagnosis no matter what the ophthalmoscopic findings may be. This rule should be
remembered.

ARTERIES: If the arteries are threadlike and
the veins normal as in Plate XVII, a diagnosis
of atrophy can be positively made without taking
the field; but it is wise to do so in all suspicious
cases.

PROGNOSIS: Very grave; vision usually totally
destroyed in time.

TREATMENT: Salvarsan or mercury and large
doses of potassium iodide may be tried. Strychnia is recommended, but treatment is usually of
little avail.

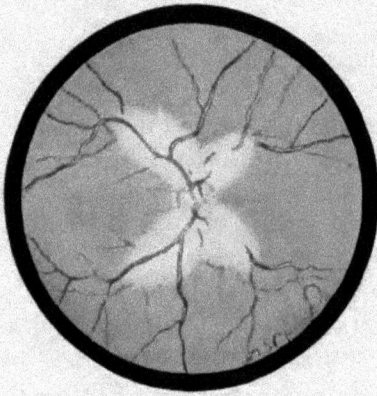

Opaque Nerve Fibres

PLATE XIX.

OPAQUE NERVE FIBRES: Plate XIX. This picture is shown in order to describe opaque nerve fibres which, while they are of no significance, should be recognized when seen, so that they should not be mistaken for some pathological condition.

The white opaque nerve fibres usually follow the principal retinal arteries. This is a normal condition of the fundus of rabbits and is not infrequently met with in man.

In the human eye however, so typical a picture as is here shown is not frequently observed; more often the condition is present only in one or two areas adjacent to the nerve head where the vessels are covered by the opaque nerve fibres.

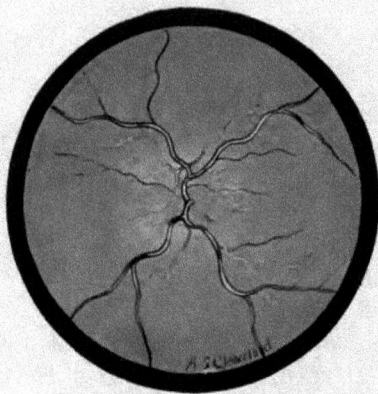

Plain Choked Disc

PLATE XX.

CHOKED DISC: Plate XX. The nerve head is swollen and the diagnosis can be made positively because when the fundus is examined, the refraction is found to be higher at the nerve head than away from it.

HYPERMETROPIC NERVE: The student is cautioned to measure the refraction of the fundus in all cases at about one diameter of the nerve head from the nerve and when this is done, to measure it at the edge of the nerve head. If the latter be more hypermetropic than the other parts of the fundus, a diagnosis of choked disc may be positively made.

It is important that the practitioner make a diagnosis of choked disc early because it is then usually amenable to treatment; and if not properly treated, optic atrophy and blindness may follow. If the choked disc is only in one eye the cause may be found in the sinuses; but if in both eyes the cause must be looked for in the cranial cavity.

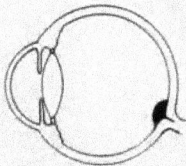

Fig. 13. Choked Disc.
Cross section Plate XX.

Figure 13 represents a cross section of Plate XX. The swelling of the nerve head can be readily seen.

PROGNOSIS: Favorable, unless from malignant tumor of the brain.

TREATMENT: If the condition is unilateral, which rarely occurs, very often appropriate sinus treatment will effect a cure. If bilateral and due to tumor of the hypophysis, the gland should be removed. Usually however, the treatment offering the greatest hope of benefit is the administration of salvarsan or mercury with large doses of potassium iodide.

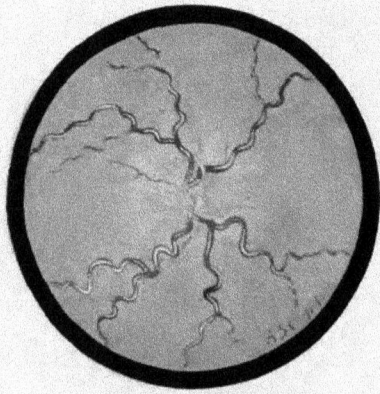

Neurorentinitis

PLATE XXI.

NEURORETINITIS: Plate XXI.   The only difference between this picture and Plate XX, is the twisting of the retinal vessels and more swelling of the optic nerve.   The nerve head is swollen and the retinal vessels are tortuous.   The diagnosis is that of a lesion both of the optic nerve and the retina (NEURORETINITIS).

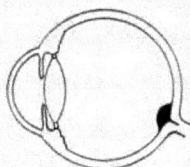

Fig. 14.   Choked disc.   Cross section Plate XXI.

Figure 14 represents a cross section of Plate XXI.   The diagnosis is readily made from the swelling of the nerve and the twisting of the retinal vessels.

PROGNOSIS: Is the same as in Plate XX.

TREATMENT: Is the same as in Plate XX.

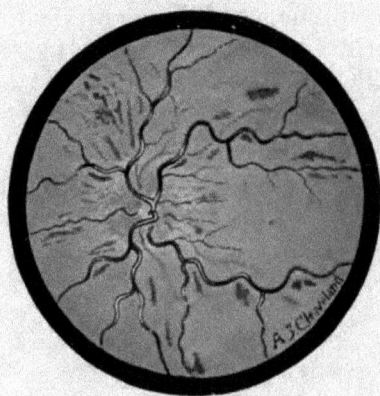

Papillitis Haemorrhagica

PLATE XXII.

PAPILLITIS HEMORRHAGICA: Plate XXII. The nerve head is swollen, the retinal vessels are twisted as in Plate XXI and the fundus is studded with hemorrhages some of which are lighter than others, indicating their more recent occurrence.

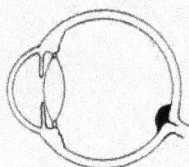

Fig. 15. Papillitis Hemorrhagica. Cross section Plate XXII.

Figure 15 represents a cross section of Plate XXII. If the media are clear, a diagnosis can readily be made and the amount of swelling of the nerve can be readily measured with the ophthalmoscope.

PROGNOSIS: Is the same as in Plate XX.

TREATMENT: Is the same as in Plate XX.

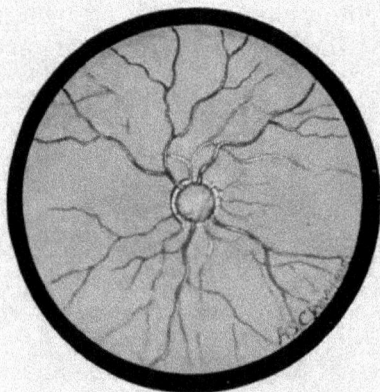

Glaucoma

PLATE XXIII.

GLAUCOMA: Plate XXIII. The retinal vessels are normal in size but they do not emerge from the center of the nerve as in normal eyes, (Plates 1 and 11) but seem to stop and disappear at the edge of the nerve head.

If the eye is refracted, the bottom of the cup or center of the nerve head will be found to be more myopic than the surrounding fundus. The arteries may pulsate and the field is usually contracted and to the nasal side.

In such a case the tension may be high, the cornea anesthetic, the anterior chamber hazy and shallow, the lens clear, the vitreous clear, but the ophthalmoscope discloses this typical picture of glaucoma.

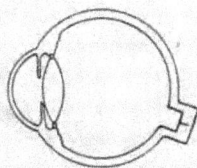

Fig. 16. Glaucoma. Cross section Plate XXIII.

Figure 16 is a cross section of Plate XXIII; there is a pushing back of the nerve head. The excavation can be as readily measured as an elevation was measured in the other plates. The difference in refraction between the normal part of the fundus and the bottom of the depression will represent the depth of the cupping.

PROGNOSIS: Guarded—see page 112.

TREATMENT: See page 112.

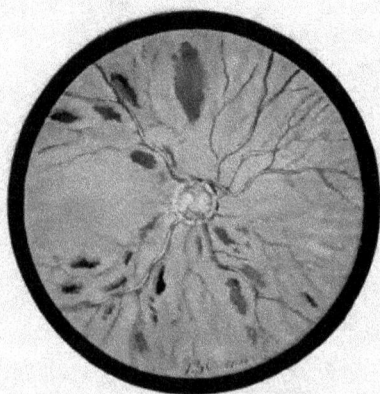

Haemorrhagic Glaucoma

PLATE XXIV.

HEMORRHAGIC GLAUCOMA: Plate XXIV. The retinal vessels are normal in size but do not emerge from the center of the optic nerve as in normal eyes. (Plates I and II.) They appear to stop at, and dip back from the edge of the optic nerve. (Plate XXIII.) The center of the optic nerve is more myopic than the normal part of the fundus and hemorrhages can be seen, some dark and some light, the latter being more recent.

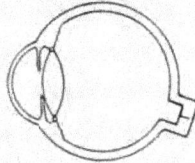

Fig. 17. Hemorrhagic Glaucoma. Cross section Plate XXIV.

Figure 17 represents a cross section of Plate XXIV: the cupping can be readily measured as in Plate XXIII.

PROGNOSIS: Grave. See page 112.

TREATMENT: See page 112.

FIELD OF VISION

Direct and Indirect Ophthalmoscopy

CHAPTER V.

THE FIELD OF VISION: The field must be studied in connection with ophthalmoscopy, because some diseases of the fundus that at first seem obscure, are made perfectly clear when the field is considered; and there are some diseases that are impossible to diagnose without the taking of the field.

WITHOUT A PERIMETER: The first thing to do in taking the field without a perimeter will be to take a small piece of paper, one quarter of an inch square, red on one side and white on the other. Hold it in front of the patient by inserting it between the points of a pen (Fig 18) and see if he is color blind.

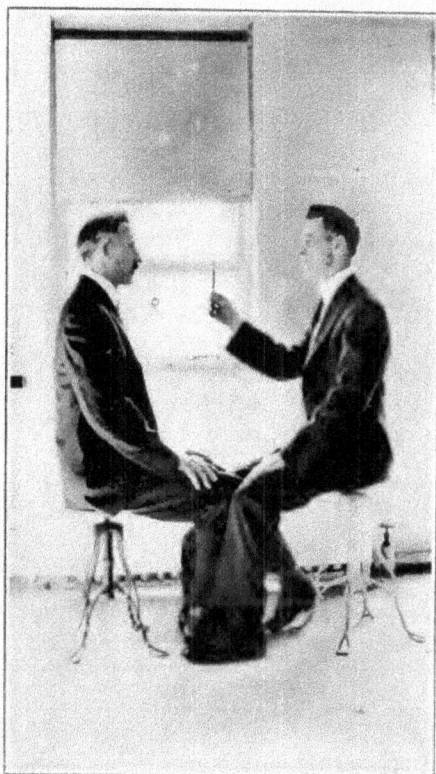

Fig. 18. Testing field for colors

CENTRAL SCOTOMA FOR RED: The examiner rotates the penholder and the red and white are alternated. When the patient looks directly at the paper he is instructed to cover one eye and look into the examiner's eye with the other. If the red color does not appear red when placed in his direct vision, or between the examiner's eye and that of the patient, and does seem so to him when the paper is moved away from the center of his field, he has a central scotoma for red.

TREATMENT: Remove the cause which is usually alcohol or tobacco and give eliminatives and 1/30 grain sulphate of strychnine qid.

If there is no central scotoma for red, next determine the extent of the fields for the various colors by comparison with your own.

To test the right eye, the patient is placed in such a position that his eyes will be on a level with the examiner's eyes; and the light from the window will fall equally on his right and on the examiner's left side. The examiner's right and the patient's left eye should be closed and both should look steadily at the pupil of the other. (Figure 19). The positions are reversed for examination of the left eye, in order that proper illumination may be obtained.

Figure 19. Comparison of Examiner's and Patient's fields. A piece of paper, red on both sides and one-quarter inch in diameter is now inserted into the pen. This paper should be moved in a plane midway between the examiner's eye and that of the patient, the examiner and patient looking into each other's eyes. Both

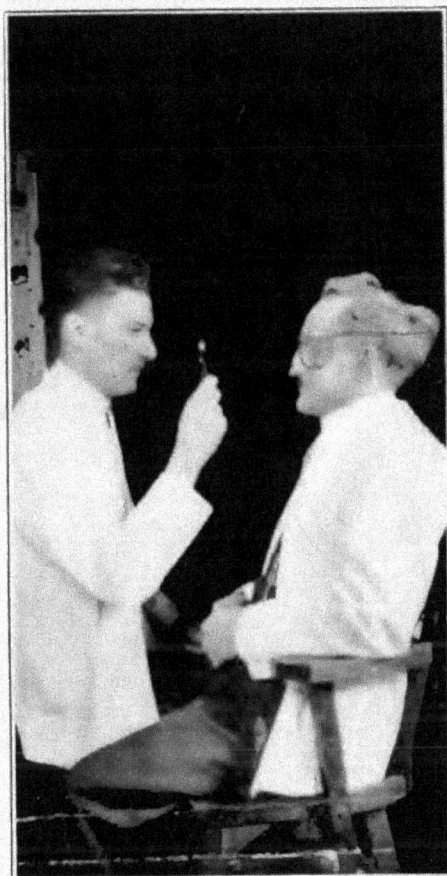

Fig. 19.   Taking field without Perimeter

should see the paper and distinguish its color about the same time if both have normal fields.

This can be done with white as well as with all the colors and, if the field is carefully taken, the student will be able to detect any deviation from the normal.

WITH PERIMETER: If the field seems suspicious with this examination, it should be taken with the perimeter (Figure 20 and 21) or with the campimeter (Figure 22).

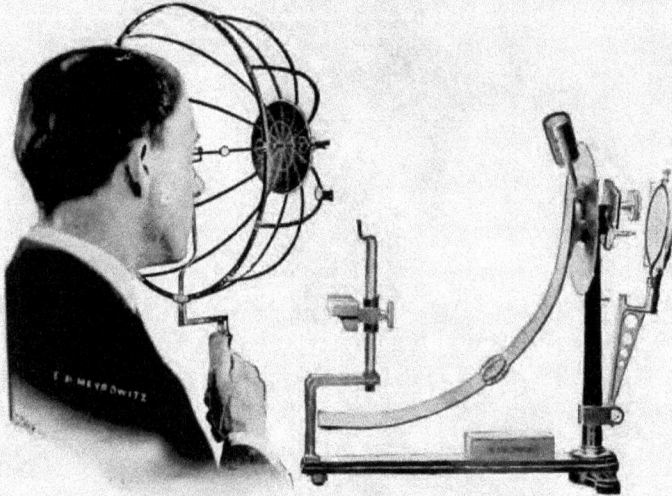

Fig. 20.   Perimeter (Meyrowitz).   Fig. 21.   Perimeter (Geneva).

A number of abnormal fields that are typical of the conditions in which they are found are inserted for the consideration of the student and that he may properly appreciate them a normal field is shown.

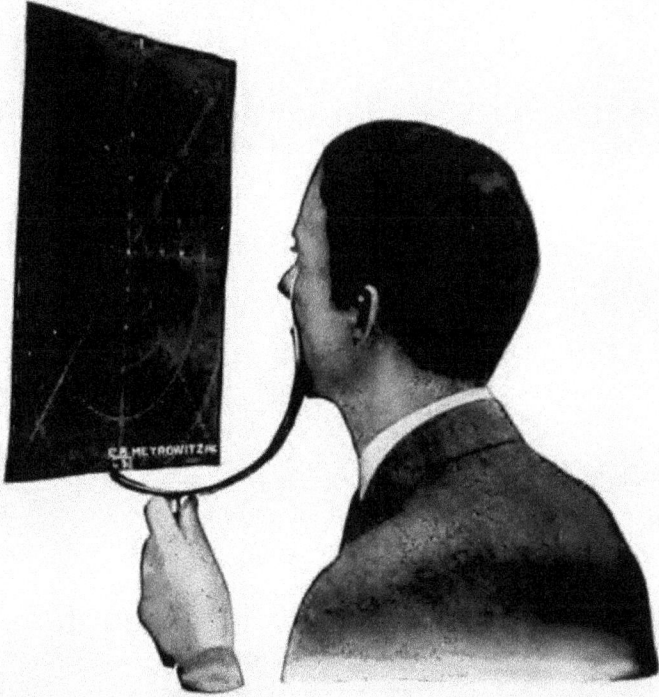

Fig. 22. Campimeter

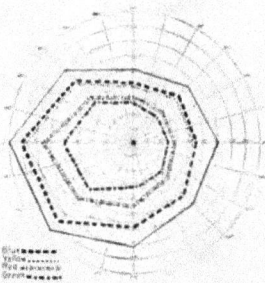

Fig. 23. Normal Field (Jennings)

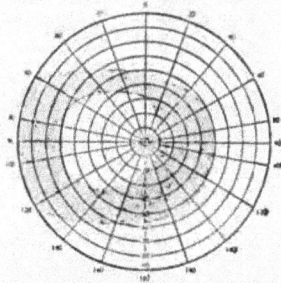

Fig. 24. The field of vision in
Glaucoma. Left eye. Peripheral
contraction especially on the nasal
side. (May)

He will note especially the extent of the individual fields for the various primary colors tested for. All of which were tested with discs ¼ inch in diameter.

GLAUCOMA: The field is contracted below and to the nasal side.

For prognosis and treatment see page 112.

OPTIC ATROPHY: The field is concentrically contracted for white and colors.

Prognosis: Grave.

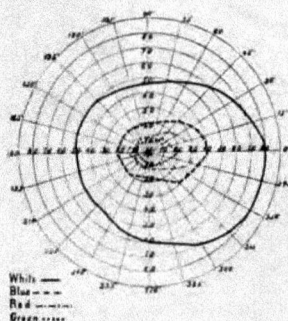

Fig. 25. Field of vision of the right eye in a case of optic-nerve atrophy. The white field is slightly contracted, the color fields markedly restricted. (deSchweinitz)

Treatment: Mercury and Iodide of Potassium should be given a trial. Strychnia is also recommended.

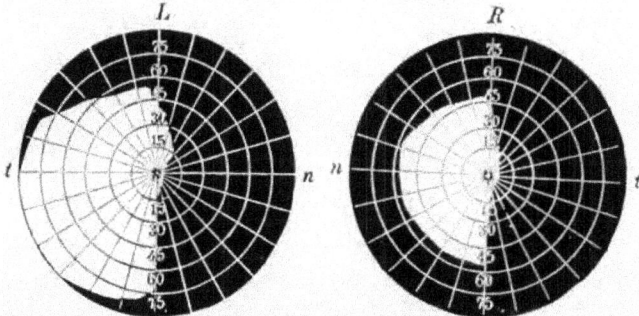

Fig. 26 and 27. Homonymous Hemiopia (Schweigger)

HEMINOPSIA: Fig. 26 and Fig. 27. The fields are entirely cut off on one side.

Fields in right homonymous heminopsia.

PROGNOSIS: Fields usually remain unchanged.

TREATMENT: If specific, salvarsan, mercury and large doses of iodide of potassium. If in elderly patients and of unknown causation, give fifteen grains of the latter four times daily.

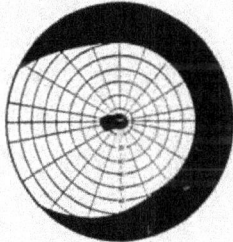

Fig. 28. Field in Toxic Amblyopia. (Fuchs)

RETROBULAR NEURITIS: TOXIC AMBLYOPIA: There is a spot in the center of the field where the patient cannot recognize the color of a small piece of red paper—central scotoma for red.

Figure 28. Field in Retrobular Neuritis.

PROGNOSIS: Good if treated early.

TREATMENT: Remove the cause which is usually tobacco or alcohol or both and give strychnia per mouth or hypodermically.

HYSTERIA: The fields overlap, that is, the green which usually lies wholly within that for the red is found to be larger and overlapping it in places. It also changes at different examinations or even when successively taken at the same sitting. When the field is being taken, even if carefully done, it will appear to change. The following two very different fields were secured by a careful operator within an hour on a patient with a well authenticated diagnosis of hysteria.

Figure 29. Field in Hysteria. Figure 30. Field in the same case one hour later. Such a variation would not occur in other diseases, and the general practitioner should understand this important condition.

PROGNOSIS: Good. However, the patient will often complain that the vision is much impaired or even sometimes claim nearly complete blindness.

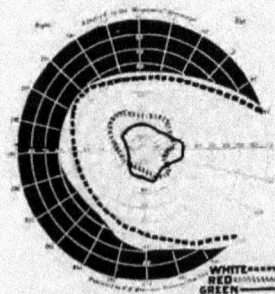

Fig. 29. Field in Hysteria   Fig. 30. Field in Hysteria

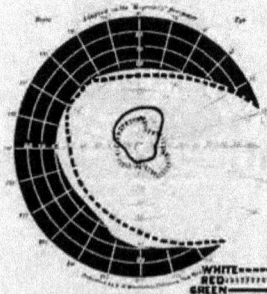

TREATMENT: Prescribe the proper glasses for the correction of any refractive error found, and give the general treatment indicated for this condition. Some placebo may be dropped into the eyes as for instance, sodii biboratis gr. V to oz. one every three hours.

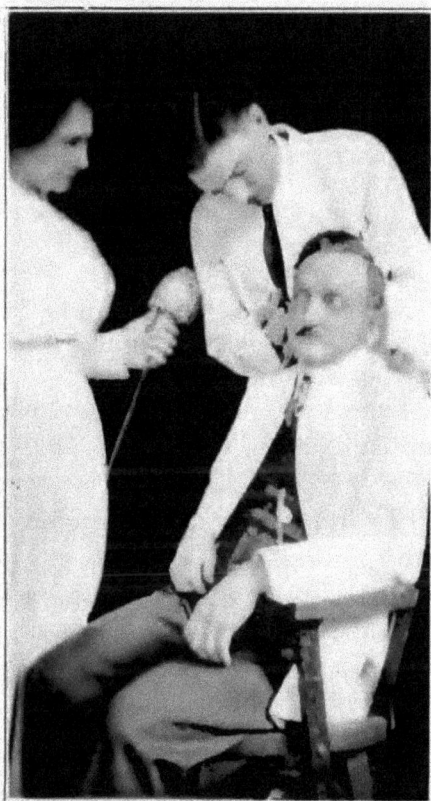

Fig. 31. Oblique Illumination

SYSTEMATIC EYE EXAMINATION: When the student has mastered the schematic eye, he will be prepared to examine a patient; but it is unwise to attempt to do so until he finds the schematic eye easy to examine, even with a small pupil and has mastered the technique of oblique illumination which he will find useful in all cases as well as ophthalmoscopy.

OBLIQUE ILLUMINATION: Condensing lens used in indirect ophthalmoscopy. Illumination of the part under inspection by means of a strong convex lens. By this means, the illumination is markedly increased and minute details are made visible. This method of examination is always used for searching for foreign bodies upon or in the cornea.

LIGHT: The source of light can be from a gas, kerosene, candle or electric light, with a frosted globe or the light from a window. The condensing lens used in connection with direct ophthalmoscopy can be used for condensing the rays of light.

INDIRECT OPHTHALMOSCOPY

When practicing indirect ophthalmoscopy (Figure 32) the patient is requested to look beyond the student's right ear when the right eye is examined, or left ear if the left eye is examined; the light is reflected into the eye from a distance of about twenty inches with the mirror of the ophthalmoscope tilted towards the light in the same manner as in the study of the schematic eye. A + 3 D. lens is placed in the ophthal-

moscope and a + 20 D.—that used for bifocal
examination—is held two inches in front of the
patient's eye, when an inverted picture of the
fundus will be seen in front of the + 20 D.
lens. The whole fundus can be studied in this
manner and all parts of it can be brought into

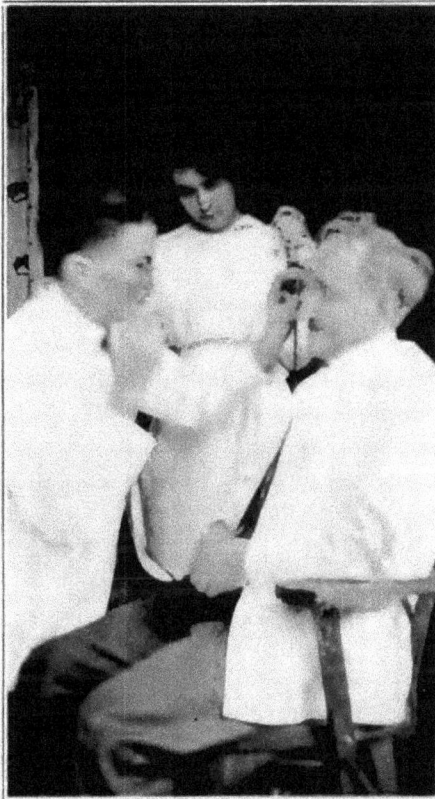

Fig. 32. Indirect Ophthalmoscopy

view by moving the + 20 D. lens from side to
side and up and down.

The indirect method is usually employed when
the eyes of children are to be examined, or when
the patient has lost the vision of one eye; and
in all other eyes where the direct method cannot
be employed.

DIRECT OPHTHALMOSCOPY. FIRST POSITION:
Figure 33. Represents the correct first position
of observer and observed in practicing direct
ophthalmoscopy. The same rules are to be observed as when the model is being used. To
examine the right eye, the light is placed on the
patient's right side on a level with his eye.

POSITION OF OBSERVER: When the right eye
is to be examined the observer sits in front and to
the right on a revolving stool that has been adjusted to the proper height. Before beginning
the ophthalmoscopic examination, the patient is
instructed to look across the room at some fixed
point and is also told to close both eyes if the
observer should get in front of him, thus keeping
him from seeing the object selected. The student
will soon learn to keep his head out of the
patient's line of vision and will readily acquire a
good position for examination.

The patient will always keep his eye quiet and
in one position if he has something for the unobserved eye to look at and he should always be
instructed to look at some selected spot before
beginning the ophthalmoscopic examination.
The mirror of the ophthalmoscope is tilted towards the light which is now reflected into the eye

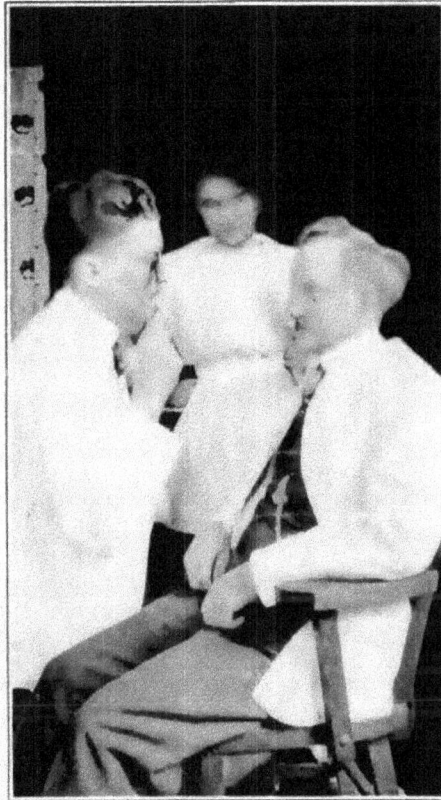

Fig. 33. Direct Ophthalmoscopy. First position

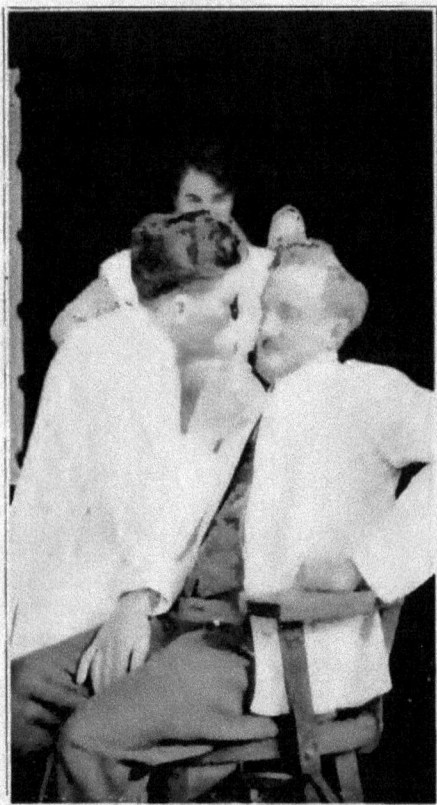

Fig. 34 Direct Ophthalmoscopy. Second position

under examination. As soon as the light is reflected into the eye, the pupil will appear red and the approach to the second position is begun.

SECOND POSITION: Figure 34. Represents the second position for direct ophthalmoscopy. The student approaches the patient from the first position and comes as close to the observed eye as possible without losing the red reflex. The student must keep both of his eyes open and relax his accommodation as much as possible by looking into the distance. If the refraction of the eye is normal or hypermetropic, the student will readily observe the retinal vessels and optic nerve when the first thing to be done before losing sight of them is to refract the eye. If the eye be myopic, the details of the fundus can be seen only with minus glasses.

LIGHT STREAKS OR WHITE LINES: It is essential to get an ophthalmoscopic picture that is not exaggerated, and to do this the student must refract the eye as he begins his ophthalmoscopic examination by looking through the aperture of the instrument. If the light streaks on the retinal vessels can be seen with the ophthalmoscope in this manner, the eye is either normal or hypermetropic.

The student should now add — 1 D. to his ophthalmoscope and, if the white lines on the arteries disappear, he will know he is dealing with a normal eye; but, if they can be seen with a + 1 D., he will know he is dealing with a hypermetropic eye and must put on stronger plus lenses until the white lines disappear. The strongest plus glass with which the light streaks or white lines can be seen *at all*, will represent the amount of hypermetropia.

If the eye is myopic, the weakest minus glass with which the white lines on the retinal vessels can be seen *at all* will represent the amount of myopia.

With these two rules in mind at all times, the student can readily detect elevations and excavations in the fundus, and, when this is done, he will be quite well prepared to make diagnosis of gross pathological lesions.

He will be able to diagnose a swelling of the nerve head, a cupping of it, or an elevation of any part of the fundus. He will also be able to tell whether spots, either white or black, are situated in the retina, in front of the retinal vessels, or in the choroid—back of them.

The student must observe the eye at close range which means that he should get as close to it as possible.

DESCRIPTION OF THE HUMAN FUNDUS: The picture of the human fundus cannot be described because of the great variations in its color. The student will observe the same general normal points as he did in the pictures in the schematic eye. He will observe the optic nerve with the retinal vessels emerging from the center of it and passing across the fundus. If the retinal vessels all stop abruptly at the edge of the disc, it is a picture of glaucoma which the student learned to recognize in the schematic eye. (Plate XXIII.)

If the retinal vessels are tortuous, a picture of retinitis will be recognized as was learned in the study of the model. (Plate XXI-XXII.) If the nerve head is more hypermetropic than the normal part of the fundus the student knows he is dealing with a case of choked disc. (Fig. 13.) All this he has learned in the examination of the schematic eye.

If some parts of the fundus are much lighter in color than others, and it is higher at the light places than at other portions, the observer will at once be suspicious of either detachment of the retina, an exudate, or sarcoma of the choroid. The student is referred to the description of these two pictures. (Plates IV and X) which are the same as the pictures of the same lesion in the human fundus.

If the student has mastered the schematic eye, he will experience no more trouble in making diagnosis of diseases of the interior of the eye than he will in making diagnosis of external diseases. Many doctors take the schematic eye too lightly and want to practice on patients before they have mastered it. Too great stress cannot be placed upon the thorough study of the schematic eye.

Ophthalmoscopy will be simplified if the human eye is not studied until the student can examine the schematic eye without any effort. If he will then begin work on patients, he will find little difficulty in getting a good view of the fundus.

The cases that appear obscure to a beginner in ophthalmoscopy usually are so because of his inability to illuminate the interior of the eye and see the pictures. If they can be seen, diagnosis will be made simple and interesting. If diagnosis of diseases of the interior of the eye is to be made simple, there is only one way to do it and that is to make ophthalmoscopy easy, which can only be done by becoming master of the ophthalmoscope upon the model.

RETINAL ARTERIES INSTEAD OF SCREEN: The student will have the retinal vessel to deal with in the human eye, and he will have lost the screen, which he has been examining in the schematic eye. He will now substitute the white streaks on the retinal arteries for the screen and examine the human eye in the same manner as he did when dealing with the model.

THE SAME TWO RULES TO REMEMBER: First, *the strongest plus lens with which he can see the white streaks on the retinal arteries AT ALL will measure the hypermetropia.* Second, *the weakest minus glass with which he can see the white streaks on the retinal arteries AT ALL will measure the myopia. THESE TWO RULES MUST BE REMEMBERED.*

DISTANCE OF EXAMINER FROM PATIENT: The examiner should get as close as possible to the eye to be examined and at the same time not to lose his light. The patient's eyes should be examined in the same manner and the same two rules observed as in the examination of the schematic eye.

WHERE SHOULD THE PATIENT LOOK: It is of the greatest importance that the patient be told to look at some point on the opposite side of the room. If the patient looks at this point and the observer sits at the side and not in front of him, he will hold the eye perfectly quiet.

If the observer gets in front of the patient and prevents him from seeing the object given him to look at, the eye that is being observed will move and the student will have difficulty in examining it; but as long as the patient has a fixed point to observe with the eye that it is not being examined there will be no difficulty.

A beginner in ophthalmoscopy should have the patient look at some object on the opposite wall and instruct him to shut both of his eyes and keep them shut, if the observer's head obstructs his vision and keeps him from seeing the object. In this manner the student will soon acquire an easy and correct position for the examination of an eye with the ophthalmoscope.

WHERE SHOULD THE EXAMINER LOOK: The examiner should keep both eyes open and imagine the picture he is examining to be twenty or more feet from him. He will in this manner learn to relax his accommodation.

ACCOMMODATION: This is a great bugbear to a beginner. He becomes confused and thinks he must be accurate in his measurements in order to be able to make diagnosis of pathological lesions. On the contrary, the principal thing necessary for him to do is to be able to recognize elevations and excavations in the back part of the eye. To do this, it is imperative that he be able to measure the refraction at some normal point, and afterward to measure it at the abnormal part without removing his eye from the ophthalmoscope or changing his position.

If the student makes a mistake in measuring the normal part of the fundus, he very likely will make the same error in measuring the abnormal part. The only necessary thing to know is the difference between the two points, and he will soon find this not at all difficult.

For instance, if the student is examining a swollen nerve, he first measures the refraction of a normal part of the fundus, usually about one diameter of the nerve head from it; he then measures that of the head of the nerve and the difference noted will represent the swelling of the nerve head.

If the normal part of the fundus as measured by the student is + 3 D. and the nerve head + 9 D., he will have 6 D. swelling. If he has made a mistake and had measured the normal part of the fundus + 6 D., would have made the same error at the nerve head and measured it a + 12. D. The difference would be the same and in either case he would have 6 D. or two millimeters of swelling of the nerve head. Other elevations would be measured in a similar manner.

EXAMINATION OF NORMAL EYES: The student should examine as many normal eyes as possible because there is no better practice with the ophthalmoscope. The principal thing for a beginner to do, when making an ophthalmoscopic examination is to measure the refraction.

He should first find the vessels in the fundus and then look for the light streaks on the retinal arteries and practice adding plus lenses in his ophthalmoscope until they disappear.

If he cannot see the light streaks on the retinal arteries and must put on minus lenses to bring them out, he is dealing with myopic eyes. He should practice putting on minus lenses to bring out the light streak on the retinal arteries remembering that the weakest one with which this can be done is the measure of the myopia.

If the student will measure the refraction in every eye he examines, he will soon be able to recognize a normal fundus; and, when this is accomplished, there will be very little trouble in detecting existing lesions.

Elevations and excavations can easily be measured when the student illuminates the interior of the eye and can measure the normal fundus. When this is accomplished, a choked disc, a glaucoma, a detached retina, an albuminuric retinitis, or a sarcoma of the choroid will be very simple matters to diagnose.

NOT NECESSARY TO REMEMBER PICTURES: It will not be necessary to remember the picture of a lesion as seen with the ophthalmoscope, but rather to know when a fundus is normal, and if abnormal, to be able to point out the abnormal points.

COLOR OF THE FUNDUS: The general background of the fundus is red but it may be very dark or it may be very light red. The retina is a transparent membrane and the color of the fundus is produced by the vascular choroid.

The normal nerve head sometimes appears red, or hyperaemic, and sometimes light, or anaemic. If the patient has normal vision, the student should not pay much attention to the color of the optic nerve; but if the vision is poor, it should be studied carefully.

OPTIC ATROPHY: In atrophy of the optic nerve, the nerve head is white or gray; but the student should never depend upon the color of the nerve head alone.

If he is suspicious of optic atrophy, the field should be taken if the patient has enough vision to make this possible. If the patient is not blind, the student can note the color of the nerve head but he can make a diagnosis of atrophy of the optic nerve by taking his field of vision long before he could be sure of such a diagnosis with the ophthalmoscope. Fields of both eyes should be taken if the patient has sufficient vision; but if one eye is blind, the field of the good one should be taken.

CHAPTER VI.

SYSTEMATIC EXAMINATION OF THE EYE

It would be impossible to make a systematic examination of the eye without a working knowledge of the ophthalmoscope; but even while we can make use of this small, inexpensive and important instrument, we have not as yet described any systematic method of examination without the careful following of which many important things would be overlooked. This systematic examination should be commenced from the front and proceed backward by certain definitely fixed steps.

FIRST STEP: INSPECTION: Figure 35. Inspection should cover all that can be seen without instruments, and a good light Fig. 35A is indispensable. The cornea is the first structure examined from front backwards. It is the seat of a great many eye affections coming under the care of general practitioners and should always receive a very careful examination for foreign bodies, ulcers and opacities.

The anterior chamber should be examined for opacities and the iris and pupil should be examined together.

The pupil should dilate when covered or protected from the light and contract to the light when uncovered or when a light is reflected into the eye. After the anterior part of the eye ball has been inspected and the tension noted (Figs. 37 and 41), the lower lid should be drawn down; the

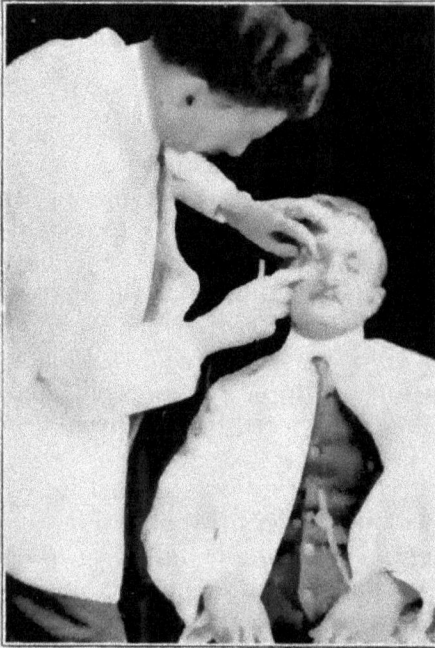

Fig. 35. Systematic Examination of the Eye

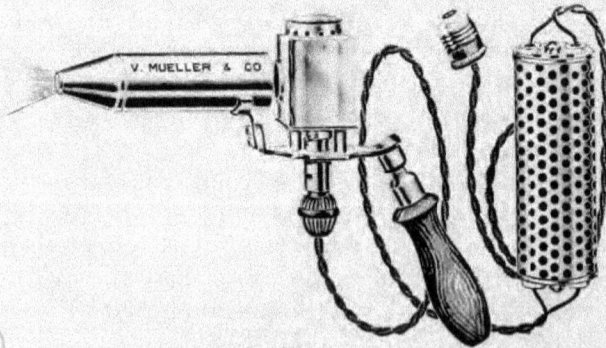

Fig. 35a. Light

conjunctiva inspected and the lachrymal sac pressed down. (Figure 36.)

If pus be pressed out of the lachrymal sac. a diagnosis of dacryocystitis will be made (Fig. 36). The upper lid should be everted for examination by drawing it downward and away from the eye and turning it over a pencil. The motility of the eyes can be observed by having the patient look up, down, right and left. If a diagnosis has not as yet been arrived at, the vision should be taken and a careful manifest refraction made.

Many doctors are satisfied with an examination less accurate than has been described, but those who can use the ophthalmoscope realize that a systematic examination has only been begun and that what is to follow, while not difficult, is of very great importance.

SECOND STEP: The patient is now taken to the dark room, and, with a + 20 D. lens that accompanies the ophthalmoscope, the light is condensed into the eye and the cornea, anterior chamber, iris, pupil and lens are again inspected: and, if the cause of the trouble be not determined, the third step should be begun.

THIRD STEP: The eye has now been examined from front backwards to the lens and we are ready for the most interesting and satisfactory part of an examination of the eyes, the use of the ophthalmoscope. The first structure to be examined in the third step is the lens. This is done with the + 16 D. of the smaller disc rotated to position behind the aperture of the instrument.

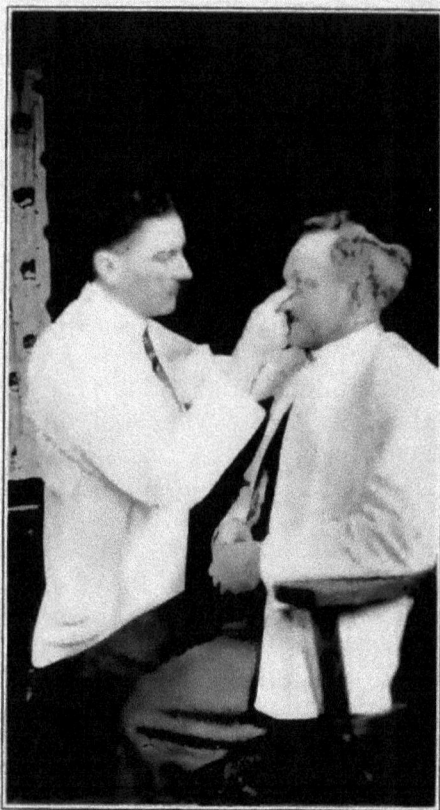

Fig. 36. Pressing upon the Lachrymal Sac.

When the ophthalmoscope is 2½ inches from
the patient's eye it will be in focus and any
opacity in the cornea, anterior chamber or lens
will appear black, because they are opaque. A
scar on the cornea that appears white by direct
inspection will appear black like a piece of steel
when seen with the ophthalmoscope.

INCIPIENT CATARACT: Beginning opacities of
the lens can be readily diagnosed with the
ophthalmoscope; and, if the diagnosis can be
made by the general practitioner, he may find
the cause of the opacity by examination of the
urine. If the physician can make a diagnosis
of beginning of cataract, he can often treat his
patient quite intelligently by giving attention to
his general condition.

If an opacity of the lens is found in a person
over forty, that is not congenital or caused by
an injury, the probability of beginning cataract
will be strong enough to warrant an examination
of the urine. If the urine is found negative, and
the vision not less than 20/40 a deep sub-conjunctival injection of 20 drops of one to 4000
cyanide of mercury is indicated, after cocainizing
and injecting 20 drops of a 2% solution of
cocain. If vision is less than 20/40, a good result
cannot be expected.

FOURTH STEP: The examination of the vitreous is made by reflecting the light into the eye
from the ophthalmoscope at a distance of two
feet from the eye and looking into the illuminated
eye through the aperture, or + 8 D. at closer
range. The patient is instructed to look up, then

down, right and left; if the vitreous is diseased, black opacities may be seen floating in it and a diagnosis of uveitis will be made. If the vitreous is clear the next step in the systematic examination should be made.

FIFTH STEP: The eye has now been examined from before backwards to and including the vitreous. The examination of the fundus should never be attempted until a systematic examination has been made of every structure in front of the retina. If this rule is observed, few mistakes in diagnosis of what is to follow will occur.

The observer should now place himself in the same position relative to the eye as was described in Figure 33; and, when in position, should instruct his patient to look at some point or spot on the opposite wall. Tell him too, that you will not obstruct the view of his object, and that if your head should get in his light, he must close both eyes and keep them closed until you tell him to open them.

RED REFLEX: The mirror of the ophthalmoscope is now tilted toward the light which is reflected into the eye at a distance of about two feet. As soon as the student reflects the light into the pupil, the red glow is seen and he approaches the eye as quickly as possible, without allowing the light to get out of the pupil. (Figure 34.)

WHITE LINE: The student while approaching the eye and through the examination, keeps both eyes open. If the eye is normal or emmetropic, the white lines in the arteries disappear when a plus lens is placed behind the aperture of the ophthalmoscope. If the white lines on the arteries are seen when a plus lens is placed behind the aperture, the eye is hypermetropic and the strongest plus glass with which the white lines can be seen *at all* indicates the hypermetropia.

If the white lines on the arteries cannot be seen when looking through the aperture of the ophthalmoscope nor when plus lenses are placed behind it, but do become visible when minus lenses are used, the weakest one with which they can be seen at all on the retinal vessels represents the degree of myopia.

RETINAL VESSELS: When measuring the refraction of the eye, the character of the retinal vessels should be noted. If the veins are normal and the arteries are small and threadlike, there is a strong suspicion of optic atrophy and the field should be taken. (See Plate XVIII.)

If the retinal vessels are twisted or tortuous, a diagnosis of retinitis will be made. (See Plate XXI.)

NERVE HEAD: If the nerve head is higher or more hypermetropic than the normal part of the retina, a diagnosis of optic neuritis will be made. (See Plate XXI and XXII.)

OPTIC NERVE: If the retinal vessels do not appear to emerge from the center of the optic nerve (Plates I and II), but seem to disappear abruptly at the edge of the nerve head, a diagnosis of glaucoma will be made. (See Plate XXIII.) However, if the optic nerve appears

white or gray, (See Plate XVIII) a diagnosis
of atrophy should not be made, until the fields of
both eyes have been taken, providing the patient
has enough vision in either eye to make this possible. The field should always be taken in all
suspicious cases.

PIGMENT: If patches of white or spots of
black are seen in the fundus, their position should
be noted. If they are on top of the retinal
vessels, Plates V and VI, the pigment must be
in the retina, but if the vessels are on top of the
spots, the lesion must be in the choroid. (Plates
XI and XII.)

If spots are found on the temporal side of
the fundus, "in the macular region" at the fovea
centralis and the patient has poor vision that
cannot be made normal with glasses, a diagnosis
of central choroiditis will be made. (Plate XIV
and XV.)

Gross lesions and changes from the normal, in
the shape of large pigmented, or atrophic spots
often appear in any part of the fundus except
the temporal side without affecting central vision.

COLOR OF FUNDUS: If some part of the fundus
is observed that is lighter in color than other
parts or is entirely without color, the normal and
abnormal portion should be refracted; and, if
the lighter part is more hypermetropic, the student knows that he is dealing with an exudate,
a detachment of the retina or a growth.

MEDIA: If the media is clear, a differential
diagnosis can readily be made. If the media is

not clear and the diagnosis with the ophthalmoscope is doubtful the tension of the eye will be
of great aid.

If the eye has been examined in the manner
described and a diagnosis cannot be made, a last
but most important step will be the taking of
the field as described on page 86.

BLOOD PRESSURE: To complete the examination the Systolic and Diastolic blood pressure
should be taken, the urine examined, and a
microscopical examination of the conjunctival
contents made if necessary.

AMBLYOPIA: It is only justifiable to make a
diagnosis of amblyopia if a diagnosis of some
other condition cannot be made.

After the student has made enough systematic
examinations to have the different steps fairly
fixed, he will not have any very great difficulty
in arriving at a proper diagnosis; and when a
diagnosis has been made, any text book on ophthalmology will give the proper treatment.

Diagnosis in ophthalmology is not difficult if
approached in the proper manner, but it would
be impossible unless the student were master of
the ophthalmoscope.

TENSION: Before taking the tension of any
eye, the patient should be requested to look
down, when we palpate by placing the tips of
two index fingers upon the upper lid and gently
press down as though palpating for pus in any
part of the body, noting the difference, if any,
in the tension of the two eyes. (Figure 37.)

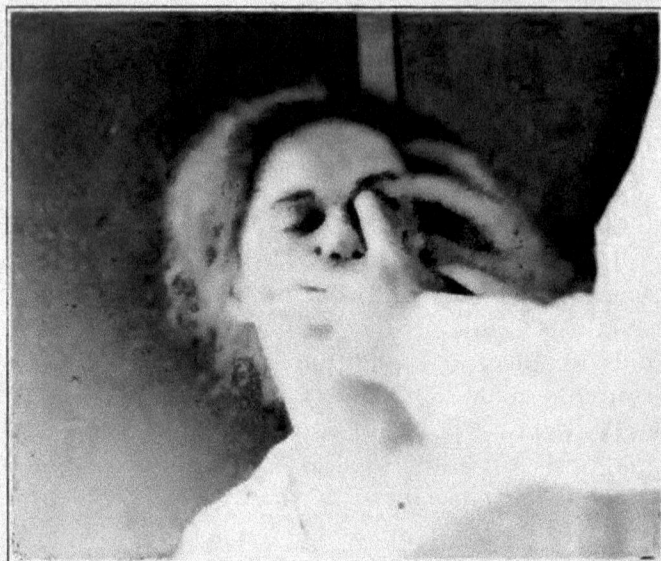

Fig. 37. Testing Tension of the Eyeball

Taking the tension with the fingers usually suffices when the eye is very soft or hard, but if a suspicion of an increase of tension exists, the tonometer should be used.

The use of the tonometer requires delicate technique; it need not be confined to an expert, but with a little practice can be of value in the hands of any general practitioner.

Before using the tonometer, the eye must be anesthetized by dropping 3 or 4 drops of a 1% solution of holocain hydrochlorate into it. Three minutes after the medicine has been instilled the patient is placed upon the table and instructed to look at the ceiling with both eyes.

The lids are kept apart with the fingers, or with Fisher's lid hooks. (Figures 39 and 40.) The tonometer is placed exactly upon the center of the cornea, held straight up, and the tension of the eye can be read from the scale on top of the instrument. (Figure 38.) The tension should be taken with one weight, then registered, and with two weights and registered, then taken again with three weights. The three readings should be the same if the instrument has been properly used. If the tonometer registers above 28, the tension is supposed to be above normal. After the three readings are registered they may be added and divided by three to get an average.

The student is again reminded that the tension is only one symptom and the vision and especially the field should always be studied in connnection with glaucoma.

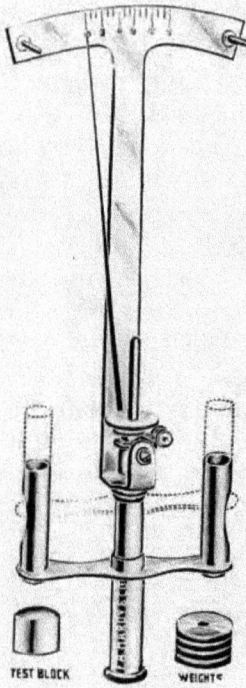

TEST BLOCK　　WEIGHTS

Fig. 38. Tonometer

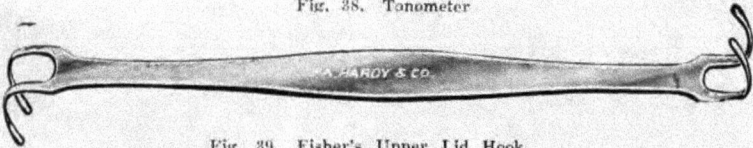

Fig. 39. Fisher's Upper Lid Hook

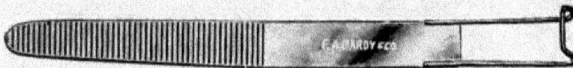

Fig. 40. Fisher's Lower Lid Hook

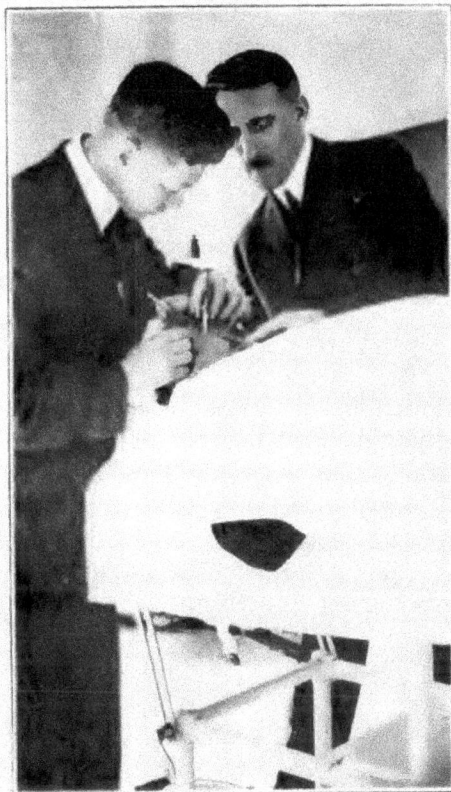

Fig. 41. Tonometer and Patient

CHAPTER VII

GLAUCOMA

The general practitioner can give his glaucoma patients proper treatment providing he can make a diagnosis; but a diagnosis is often impossible without a working knowledge of the ophthalmoscope.

The symptoms of glaucoma are unlike those of any other disease and they are usually so well marked that a diagnosis is within the grasp of the general practitioner.

If a systematic examination of the eye is made (see Page 97) it will not be difficult to make a diagnosis of glaucoma if it exists; and all that appears necessary to enable the general practitioner to make such a diagnosis, is to have an ophthalmoscope, a perimeter, and a tonometer and to know how to use them.

Clinically, glaucoma is a simple proposition, but scientifically much is to be learned. The subject will be treated clinically in the hope that general practitioners will be able to make a diagnosis. Only two varieties of glaucoma need be mentioned, glaucoma which is the result of some unknown cause; and glaucoma which is caused by some known disease, injury, or operation upon the eye ball.

SYMPTOMS: A patient usually over forty, complaining of some loss of vision, pain in the eyes or head, observing a picture of a rainbow around the light, should be looked upon as a possible case of glaucoma.

At this particular point the author believes it desirable to simplify the subject by omitting the word glaucoma and substituting the words "Plus tension." Any eye that has tension above normal is glaucomatous; and when the tension is above normal, it must be reduced in some manner because of the danger of loss of vision.

CAUSE OF PLUS TENSION: Injuries to the eye or operations upon the eye ball and inflammation of the eye causing adhesions of the iris to the lens cause many eyes to become hard, or have plus tension; but plus tension may appear and destroy the eye without any known cause.

Examination of the eye from before backward in a typical case would be as follows:

PLUS TENSION: Cornea anesthetic and hazy; anterior chamber shallow; aequeous, cloudy, iris muddy; pupil dilated; lens clear; vitreous clear; pulsating retinal arteries; nerve head cupped.

(See Plates XXIII and Figure 16.) Field contracted below and to the nasal side. (Figure 24.)

All of these symptoms need not be found, but enough of them to establish a diagnosis can usually be found in glaucoma.

If the student is doubtful about any increase in tension such as is usually determined by the fingers. (Figure 37) he can measure the tension with the tonometer which is more dependable, especially to the inexperienced, in taking the tension (Figure 38); and, if still in doubt, the field can be taken with the perimeter which is all important and does not require an expert.

If all these precautions are taken in doubtful cases, the medical men would not make many errors in diagnosing. When the condition has been diagnosed in the eye complained of, taking the tension and field of the other eye is imperative. The prompt institution of treatment in this incipient stage often arrests the progress of the disease.

PROGNOSIS: The prognosis will depend upon the cause, being grave, in those that have no known causation, as in Plate XXIII and XXIV, but guarded in all cases.

TREATMENT: In those that have plus tension from injuries to or operations upon the eye ball, or inflammations that have caused adhesions of the iris to the lens, atropin sulphate is indicated, using two drops of a 1% solution dropped into the eye three times a day; always instructing the

patient to press upon the tear duct for a minute
after putting in the drops.

In those that have plus tension from some unknown cause, the treatment is quite simple and
consists of a solution of eserin salicylate to be
dropped into the eye instead of atropin.

As soon as the eye is found to have tension
above the normal without a known cause for the
condition, two drops of freshly prepared and
sterile solution of salicylate of eserin should be
instilled into the eye every three hours day and
night. The medicine needs to be continued
throughout the entire twenty-four hours because
the effect of eserin lasts only about three hours.

It is often best to begin with a solution of
1_2 grain to the ounce. If the tension is reduced
to normal with this weak solution, it can be kept
up indefinitely; or a solution of nitrate of pilocarpin, "Posey" can be substituted for the eserin
to be used during the day with eserin at night.
If the weak solution does not have any effect
upon the tension after three instillations, the
strength should be made one grain to the ounce.
If this strength does not suffice with three instillations, a still further increase can be made up to
four grains to the ounce unless it causes severe
pain. Eserin and Pilocarpin are both used at
the same time by some with good effect.

Some insist upon the patient being in bed while
the myotic is being used. A general examination
should be made in an endeavor to locate the cause
which should include the examination of the urine,
blood, mouth, throat, nose and intestinal canal

with an X-Ray of the teeth, and such general treatment as is indicated, including eliminatives especially (an enema should be given every night). If the tension is not reduced, operative procedure should not be delayed.

ATROPIN AND ESERIN: *The student is cautioned regarding atropin and eserin. Eserin is used in all cases where the eye has plus tension without a known cause, and atropin after injuries to the eye,* after operation upon the eye ball, *and when the eye has plus tension from inflammation where the iris is adherent to the lens.*

The student will see by the foregoing that eserin and atropin have their distinctive places. It is not often that a mistake is made—because of the exact indications for the use of each.

OPERATIVE TREATMENT: When an eye is injured, the lens may become opaque. "Traumatic Cataract," produces swelling; and, in patients over twenty, it is often necessary to remove the lens. In such cases, atropin or eserin would not suffice because the swollen lens would be the cause of the plus tension and its removal would be the only rational method of reducing it.

OCCLUDED PUPIL.: Adhesions of the iris to the lens resulting from inflammation of the eye sometimes prevent the aqueous from passing from the anterior to the posterior chamber and may be so firm that they cannot be broken by the use of atropin. They may thus be the cause of the increased tension.

In such a case an iridectomy should be done upward to reduce the tension without disfiguring

the eye, since the iridectomy would be covered by
the lid. It is not necessary to make a deep
iridectomy for this purpose as must be done for
reducing tension with an unknown cause.

PARACENTESIS: A cataract knife is passed into
the anterior chamber, turned slightly upon its
edge, the anterior chamber slowly evacuated, the
knife carefully withdrawn, and the eye bandaged.
Various operative procedures have been devised
for reducing the tension when the cause is not
known but commonly called glaucoma: a properly performed iridectomy has produced the best
results in the author's hands and the Smith
method has been unusually satisfactory.

CHAPTER VIII

OPTICAL PRINCIPLES, TEST TYPE, LENSES, REFRACTION AND CYLOPEGICS

Each of the various methods of diagnosis of refractive errors is some application of the use of lenses; and the placing of them before the defective eye for more or less constant wear is the only means we have for their correction. It is therefore necessary to try to make clear the theory of their action, and their application for these purposes.

LIGHT: Light or radiant energy is given off from all luminous objects, its greatest source of course being the sun. It is transmitted by wave action in the universal ether at the enormous speed of nearly two hundred thousand miles per second through empty space where it meets with no resistance. As it approaches the earth, however, its speed is slightly reduced by the interference offered by our atmosphere and more so by other objects of greater density with which it comes in contact, and which, if at all pigmented, absorb a greater or less quantity of the light as it passes through or enters into them. The whole theory of the action of lenses rests on the above phenomena.

LAWS OF LENS ACTION: In taking up the study of the action of lenses, the student must accept the following two laws:

1. A ray of light entering and leaving a refracting medium perpendicular (or normal as it is called in optical nomenclature) to its surface, is not refracted but continues with its direction unchanged. Such a ray is spoken of as the axial ray.

2. A ray of light entering a denser from a rarer refracting medium is deviated toward the perpendicular to the entered surface; and leaving a denser to reenter a rarer medium, is refracted away from the perpendicular to the surface last passed through. Practically, however, in our work the net result of this double refraction is a deviation of the refracted ray toward the thicker portion of the denser refracting medium.

PRODUCTION OF IMAGES: The next point in our study of lens action is the consideration of the phenomena of the production of images which is really only an application of the two above laws, differing from the latter only in the fact of considering the action of all the incident rays instead of only a few.

ACTION OF CONVEX LENSES: If, in the case of the convex lens, (Figure 42) instead of only one or two incident rays, we consider the action of all the rays that enter, we can readily see that we must have such a result as is illustrated in Figure 42, in which all the incident rays are shown converging and finally coming to a point of focus after passing through the lens.

This is not a matter of theory, but can be shown experimentally with any suitable source of illumination and a screen placed at the proper distance from the lens.

When the source of illumination is placed twenty feet or farther away, usually spoken of as infinity from the lens, the rays that leave it and enter the latter, do so practically parallel to each other; and, in order to secure a distant image, which will be inverted, of the source of illumination, the screen must be placed at a certain definite distance from the center of the lens. This point is called the principal focus of the lens and its distance from the center of the latter is the focal length. This last is made use of in computing the dioptric or refractive strength of the lens as described on page 127. Since the image in this case can be demonstrated as described above, it is spoken of as a positive or real image, and the point at which it occurs as a positive or real focus.

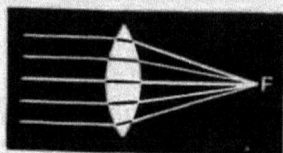

Fig. 42. The Action of a Convex Lens on Parallel Rays. (May.)   Fig. 43. The Action of a Concave Lens on Parallel Rays. (May.)

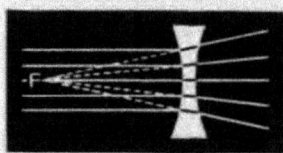

ACTION OF CONCAVE LENSES: Figure 43. When we apply the above principles to the concave lens, we secure the very different result illustrated in Figure 43.

The parallel rays entering the lens are caused to diverge and obviously can never come to a focus. However, if we place one eye in the path of these divergent rays, we are able to observe an erect reduced image of the source of illumination which is the result of the prolonging backward of the refracted divergent rays shown by the dotted lines in Figure 43; this image is located at the principal focus of the lens. Such an image which cannot be thrown on a screen and can be observed only through the concave lens producing it, is spoken of as a virtual image.

CONJUGATE FOCI: Another, but minor matter to be considered in studying the action of convex lenses is that of conjugate foci, (Figure 44) in

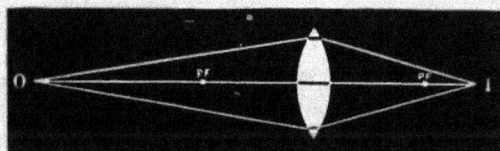

Fig 44. Conjugate Foci of a Convex Lens. (May.)

which the source of illumination being less than twenty feet away, the incident rays enter the lens not parallel to each other but decidedly diverging. Obviously they will not be brought to a focus at a point as near the lens as they would if they had entered the latter parallel to each other.

In such a case, the source of illumination and its image beyond the lens are spoken of as conjugate foci, and are interchangeable and capable of being located at any point between the principal focus of the lens and twenty feet.

THE SPECTRUM: There is, however, one strik

ing phenomena that occurs when performing the above experiment which the student should understand. If a suitable screen (a prism) be provided on which the emergent rays are allowed to fall, instead of a colorless illumination of it occurring, such as happened when the convex and concave lenses were used, there will be a beautiful display of colors always in a definite order—red, orange, yellow, green, blue, indigo and violet, reading from the apex toward the base of the prism. These colors in this order are spoken of as the primary colors of the SOLAR SPECTRUM.

CONCAVE AND CONVEX LENSES AS PRISMS: The above phenomena occur in a modified degree

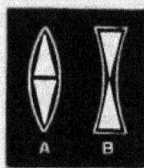

Fig. 45. Formation of Lenses by Prisms. (May.)

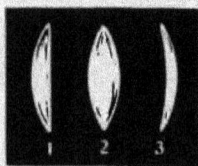

Fig. 46. Convex Lenses. 1, Plano-Convex; 2, Bi-Convex; 3, Convex meniscus. (May.)

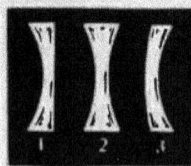

Fig. 47. Concave Lenses. 1, Plano-Concave; 2, Bi-Concave; 3, Concave meniscus. (May.)

when strong convex or concave lenses are used, since, as shown by Figure 45, they may quite properly be regarded as collections of prisms with their bases toward the center or periphery of the lens as the case may be.

The last point is aptly illustrated by the customarily used rapid method for determining the character of an unknown lens, looking at a

distant object through it while moving the lens
slightly from side to side, when it will be noted
that the object looked at seems to move in the
direction opposite to that taken by the lens if
it be convex and in the same direction if it be
concave.

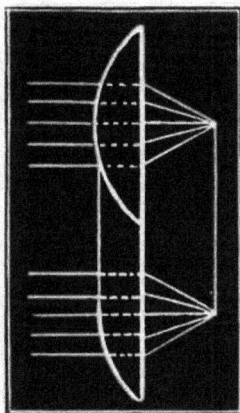

Fig. 48. Refraction by Convex   Fig. 49. Refraction by Concave
Cylindric Lens. (Ball.)   Cylindric Lens. (Ball.)

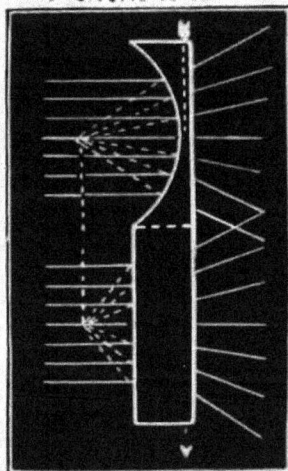

CYLINDRICAL LENSES: There remains yet another form of lens to consider, which, from its
shape, is called the cylindrical lens and which may
be either convex or concave. It differs in shape
from the other forms in, that in one direction or
axis of the lens, as it is called, there is absolutely
no curvature and hence, rays entering in this
region undergo no refraction.

On leaving the axis, however, a curvature begins and gradually increases until, in the meridian at right angles to the axis, it reaches a maximum and rays passing through it are markedly refracted.

As stated above this lens may be either convex or concave, and the phenomena of image production occurs in precisely the same way as previously described save that, instead of a focal point, a focal line is produced which always extends in the same direction as does the axis of the lens.

ACTION OF LENSES IN PRACTICE: In the above discussion of the action of lenses, which will not be referred to again but which must be thoroughly understood by the student for the purpose of emphasis and other reasons, much has been said about the focus, the focal distance, etc. In actual practice, however, in either diagnosis or treatment actual images are never produced and incident rays are never brought to a focus save in the applications of indirect ophthalmoscopy. Lenses are used rather, even on eyes from which the crystalline lens has been removed, to modify the incident rays only in an amount equal to the deficiency of the eye under examination or treatment, leaving the final focus and image to be produced by the refractive system of the eye itself.

LENS MATERIAL: A careful consideration of the above will make it clear that any transparent object with variously shaped surfaces may act in the capacity of a lens. It having been found that air having a refractive strength only slightly in excess of a vacuum, it has been taken as a

standard and experiments have been performed
with many different substances to determine their
refractive powers as compared with that of air,
the results being recorded as indices of refraction.
Those of the commoner ones and of the refractive
mediae of the eye are given in the following table:

INDICES OF REFRACTION

Air 1.00
Water 1.33
Crown glass 1.5
Flint glass 1.58
Diamond 2.4
Cornea 1.33
Aqueous humor 1.3
Crystalline lens 1.41
Vitreous humor 1.35

It is obvious that of the above substances, glass
is the only one that can be made use of on a
commercial scale for the manufacture of lenses;
and, of the two forms, crown glass has been found
to be preferable. Flint glass is made use of only
and in combination with crown glass in the manufacture of optical instruments in which spherical
aberration must be overcome, and for making
certain forms of bifocal lenses.

TEST LENS AND TRIAL FRAME: Crown glass
as noted above has been found to have certain
advantages over flint that have resulted in its
coming into general use. In addition to its use
in the various other instruments, it is made up in
sets of pairs of convex and concave spheres and

convex and concave cylinders varying in refractive strength by suitable intervals from the weakest lens used to as strong as is usually required, mounted in circular frame in the handle of which is cut a plus or minus sign to indicate the character of the contained lens, and on which is also stamped its dioptric value, of one and one-half inch, or one and one-fourth inch, of which the former has been found to be the preferable.

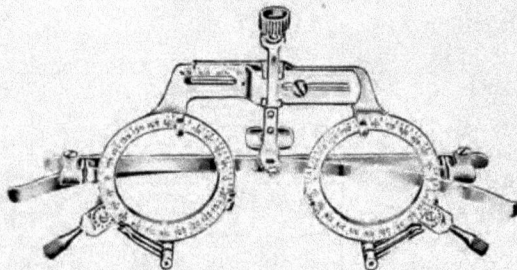

Fig. 50. Trial Frame

The trial frame should have a quadrant attached to each cell which should be capable of various adjustments in order that the lenses may be properly centered before the eyes and that it with its weight, which is necessarily considerable, may be comfortably worn. (See Figure 50.)

Various substitutes have been devised to overcome the objection to the weight of the trial frame, which occasions considerable difficulty.

Cylindrical lenses are further distinguished by having a short line etched at the extremities of the meridian of the axis, and sometimes in addi-

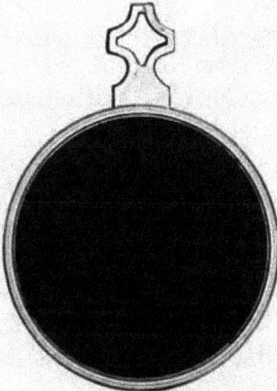

Fig. 51. Blank Disc

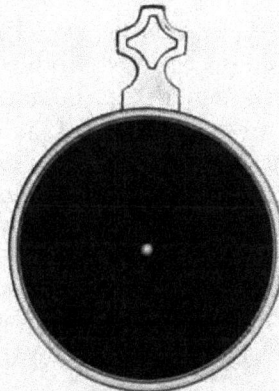

Fig. 52. Pinhole Disc

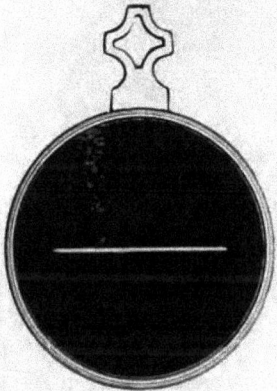

Fig. 53. Stenopic Slit

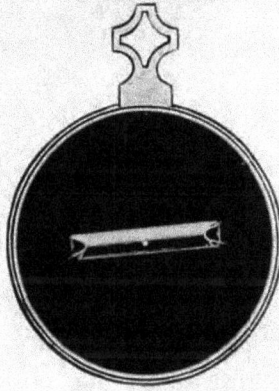

Fig. 54. Maddox Rod

tion to the above a frosting of the borders of the lens parallel to the axis. Some operators prefer a further general differentiation between the plus and minus lenses having the frames of the two forms made of different materials, as for instance, aluminic for the plus and gold plated for the minus.

ACCESSORIES AND PRISMS: In addition to the spheres and cylinders described above certain accessory discs, the uses of which will be discussed later, are provided, as well as a set of prisms with their strengths usually expressed in prism dioptres stamped on the handle.

A prism dioptre is described as the amount of prismatic effect produced by decentering a one dioptre sphere one centimeter in any direction or a one dioptre cylinder a similar distance in the direction at right angles to its axis.

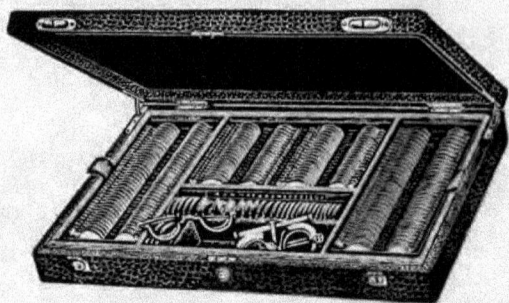

Fig. 55. Trial Case

THE TRIAL CASE: For convenience sake all of the above are collected in sets and kept in suitable containers which are made in various forms to suit the needs of the operator; of these the most common form is shown in figure 55 and the whole collection with the containers is known as the trial case.

In determining the refractive condition of an eye by the so called subjective method, the patient with the trial frame properly adjusted looks at

some object selected by the operator and reports
to the latter the effects on vision produced by the
introduction into the trial frame of various lenses
or accessories from the trial case, the successive
changes being determined by the effects produced. With the many workers in the same field
it has, of course, been found desirable to have a
standard of tests objects, as they are called. For
distant testing, Snellen's test type with its various adaptions for the examination of illiterates is
the one used. As was stated in the discussion of
lens action, after having traveled a distance of
twenty feet from their source or origin, rays of
light are practically parallel. For accurate work
this distance should be maintained either actually
or by the use of a reversed chart and a mirror
between the patient and the test type, in all distant subjective examination.

SNELLEN'S TEST TYPES: The final application
of the Snellen principle is the production of a
chart such as is shown in Figures 56, 57 and 58,
consisting of letters of such different sizes that,
conforming to the above principle and when well
illuminated, the various lines should be read by
the individual with normal vision at distances
ranging from ten to two hundred feet.

THE ILLITERATE CHART: Various modifications of this chart have been devised but the
most useful one and the only other one the
operator need have is the "E" chart, (Figure
57) for use with those who do not read English
and for children who when provided with the
metal "E," (Figure 59) become very much

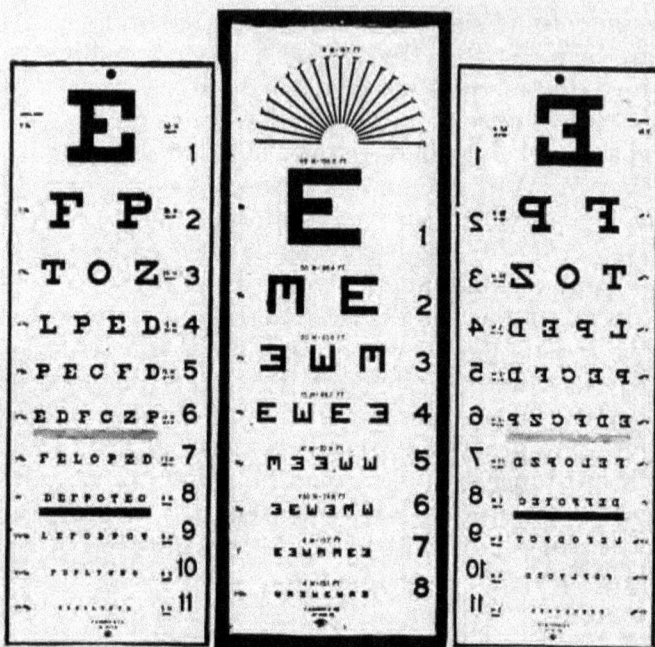

Fig. 56. Snellen Test Type.

Fig. 57. Snellen Test Type—Illiterate.

Fig. 58. Snellen Test Type — Reversed for Mirror.

interested in indicating the letters called to their attention giving more accurate answers than when one of the numerous toy charts are used.

SPECIAL CHARTS: Some operators claim there is an advantage in having the colors reversed, that is white letters on a black background, and a recent investigator has presented evidence to show that red letters on a white background give more accurate results.

THE REVERSED CHART: Should it happen that the operator is working in an office of con-

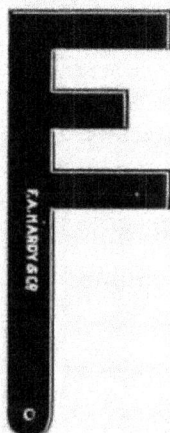

Fig. 59. Metal "E" with Handle

siderably less than twenty feet length, he will need to make use of a reversed Snellen chart. (Figure 58) hung in a good light above the patient's head and a mirror placed ten feet away which doubles the distance. If this distance does not correspond with the end of the room, the mirror may be hung on a bracket so that it may be swung out into position as needed and back against the wall when not in use. With this arrangement, one can point out letters on the chart without leaving the patient's side—really a great convenience.

TESTING AND RECORDING VISUAL ACUITY: Of course, no operator refracts patients with the chart of a distance of two hundred feet, but it is found convenient to have type that should be read up to that distance as a means of recording visual acuity. Thus, if when seated at a distance of twenty feet from the chart the patient reads the lines that should be read at that distance, his visual acuity is described as 20 20 or normal. Not infrequently persons are met with who have better than the normal visual acuity—20/15 or even 20/10, while in practice we constantly meet people with a vision of 20/200 or even less, in which last event we bring the chart nearer the patient until the largest type can be read, when we record his vision with a fraction making two hundred the denominator, and the distance at which the largest type was read the numerator; as for instance, if he read the 20/200 line at 8 feet we record his vision 8/200. In cases of very low acuity of vision, we note the distance at which the patient can count the operator's fingers in a good light and against a dark background, recording the result as "counts fingers at three feet" or 3/200, when still further reduced, we record the vision as "has perception and projection," and no vision being present, "has no perception or projection," perception meaning simply sensitiveness to light and projection the ability to determine from what direction it comes.

JAEGER'S TEST TYPE:. For testing and recording the near vision and in its correction when necessary Jaeger's test type, which consists of different sizes of ordinary Roman types arranged in order of size and numbered, beginning with the finest as Jaeger one (abbreviated J. 1. etc.) Figure 60 is used.

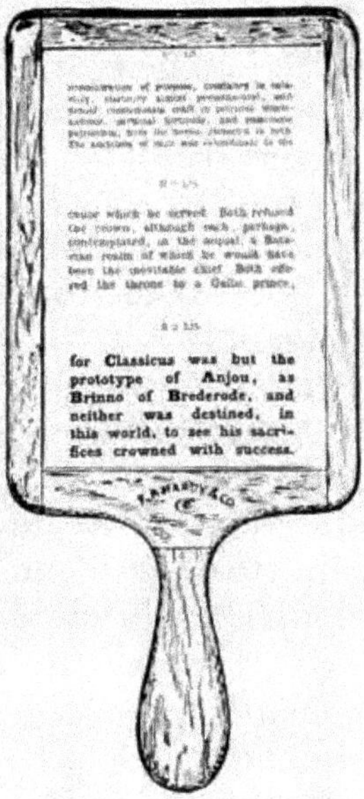

Fig. 60. Jaeger Test Type

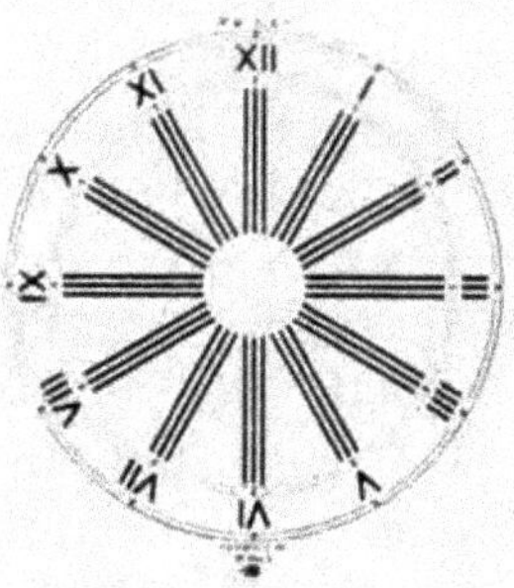

Fig. 61. Astigmatic Chart

Of recent years, a new system of numbering the Jaeger type has come into use, the application of which will be discussed under presbyopia.

THE ASTIGMATIC CHART: In addition to the above charts another, the so-called astigmatic chart, has been devised of which many forms are in use, the commonest one perhaps being illustrated in Figure 61.

While some operators consider its use indispensable in the correction of astigmatism, others prefer to dispense with it and to depend on visual results, as determined with the Snellen type, alone in their work with the trial case.

THE USE OF THE TRIAL CASE: When one is familiar with lenses and their action, he is ready to consider their application in the diagnosis of refractive errors. The use of the trial case and the test charts for this purpose is often spoken of as manifesting or taking the manifest since it is most frequently done without the ciliary muscle having been put at rest. If this latter has been done, we speak of refracting under a cyclopegic or taking the static refraction subjectively.

RULES: In either event, accurate results are dependent upon a systematic use of the test lenses and accessories, the rules for which must be learned and followed, and which will now be set forth:

1st. The patient must be comfortably seated twenty feet from the well-illuminated Snellen chart with the trial frame adjusted so as to be comfortable and with the centers of the lens cells before the pupils of his eyes.

2nd. The left eye being covered with the blank disc Figure 51, note and record the acuity of vision of the right eye.

3rd. Now insert in the trial frame a $+.50$ D. sphere. If improvement occur, or if there be no impairment, gradually increase the plus until the addition of a $+.25$ sphere causes an impairment of the best vision thus far secured.

4th. Having secured all the improvement possible with plus spheres, or, if they have been rejected, and with the sphere in position if used, insert a $+ .50$ D. cylinder with the axis at various positions; and, if improvement occurs at any point in the rotation, select the point of greatest improvement as the proper position for the axis and increase the strength of the cylinder so long as there is improvement. *Put on all the plus sphere or cylinder, that the patient will accept without blurring the smallest letters he can read.*

5th. If plus spheres and cylinders have been rejected, exhibit a — .50 D. sphere, and, if improvement occurs, increase cautiously as long as improvement occurs taking care not to over correct, (a very easy thing to do when minus lenses are accepted) because with many people greater acuity of vision is secured when the accommodation is brought slightly into play.

6th. If minus spheres have not produced a visual acuity equal to that obtained with the pin hole, exhibit a — .50 D. cylinder with its axis at various positions; and, if improvement occurs at any position, select the point of greatest improvement as the proper position for the axis and increase the strength of the cylinder cautiously as long as improvement occurs taking care not to over correct.

USE AS LITTLE MINUS SPHERE OR CYLINDER AS POSSIBLE

7th. *Crossed Cylinders:* If an improvement, but not normal vision or vision equal to that obtained with the pin hole, has been secured with a plus cylinder, try the cautious exhibition of minus cylinders in combination with the plus with the axis at right angles to that of the latter.

8th. When normal vision has not been secured with lenses insert the pin hole disc (Figure 52) and note if there be further improvement, in which event, it will usually be possible to secure an equal vision with lenses.

9th. Do not hurry or be peremptory with a patient; while it is inadvisable to ask leading questions, patience and tact while using the trial case will usually be repaid by greater accuracy of results.

FOGGING: The so called fogging system consists in placing a + 6.D. in front of the eye under examination, producing a strong artificial myopia with a great reduction of vision.

A — 1.D. is placed in front of the + 6.D., then a — 2.D. and so on down until the best vision is produced by the minus glass. If vision is then abnormal, a minus cylinder is placed in front of the minus sphere turning the cylinder in the trial frame until the clearest axis is found, and adding cylinders at this axis until the best vision is obtained. The minus glass is not removed from the + 6.D. until the next stronger minus glass is in place.

The fogging method, building down from a + 6.D. gives the same prescription or result to the author as building up with weak + glasses described on page 132.

The following illustrations from Dr. Carl Wagner of Chicago, gives a good description of the fogging system. (Pages 138-153.)

Fig. A.   Fig. B.

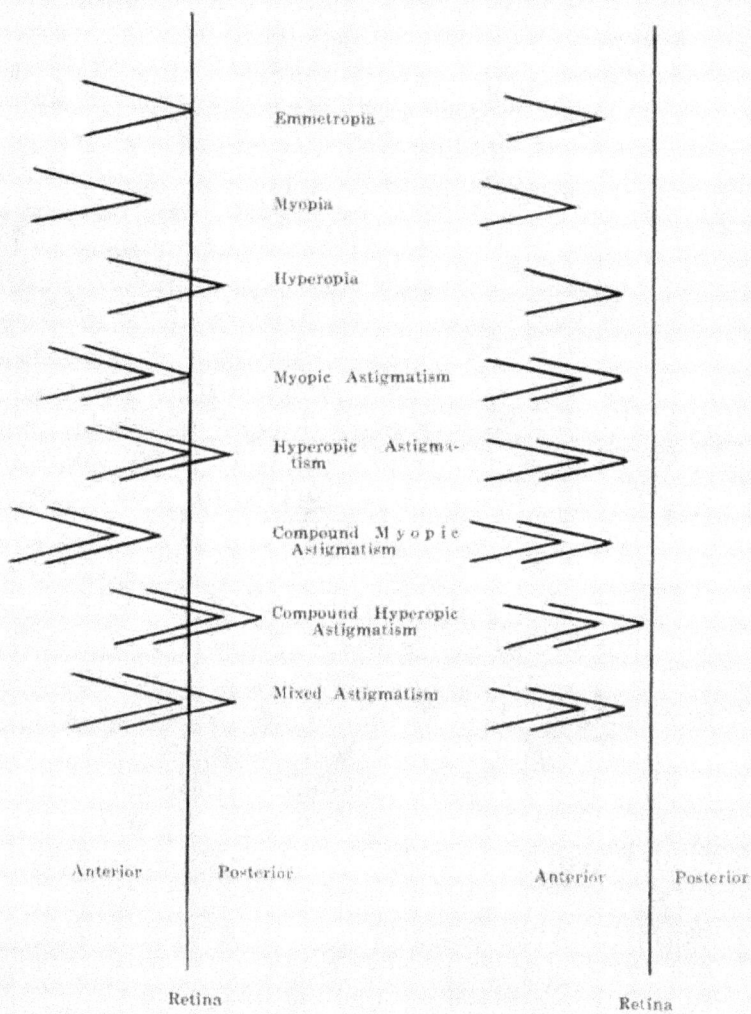

Emmetropia

Myopia

Hyperopia

Myopic Astigmatism

Hyperopic Astigmatism

Compound Myopic Astigmatism

Compound Hyperopic Astigmatism

Mixed Astigmatism

Anterior   Posterior   Anterior   Posterior

Retina   Retina

Fig. 62.

Fig. A (62) shows the foci of the various errors of refraction, and their relative position to the Retina.

Fig. B (62) shows the position of the foci after a + 6.D. sph. has been placed in front of each error.

Figures 63 and 64 show Hyperopic and Myopic Astigmatism. Assuming the amount of error in both instances to be 2.D., and the best obtainable vision to be 20 40, we may, in each case, through the use of a + 6 D. sphere, bring the focus far in front of the fundus, the resulting vision then being much below 20 40. In order to regain this 20/40 in Figure 63, it is necessary to reduce the + 6 D. sphere, by the gradual application of weaker lenses, and it will invariably be found that this is finally accomplished through the use of a + 2 D. sphere, when both foci will be in position as in Figure 64.

In order to obtain 20/40 in Figure 64, we further reduce the strength of the lenses, until 0 is reached, at which time with no lens in the trial frame, the foci would again be in the same relative position as they were.

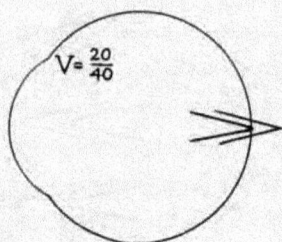

Fig. 63

In correcting the astigmatism, an attempt must be made, through the use of spherical lenses, to obtain as good or better vision than that which exists in the un-aided eye.

When the result is obtained, it becomes the key to further proced-ure. Leaving the ac-complishing lens in the trial frame, minus cyl-inder lenses are now used to complete the astigmatic correction.

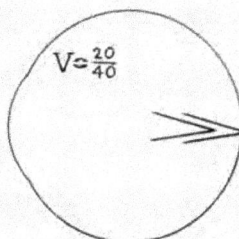

Fig. 64.

Experimental Correction of a Normal Eye. (EMMETROPIA.)

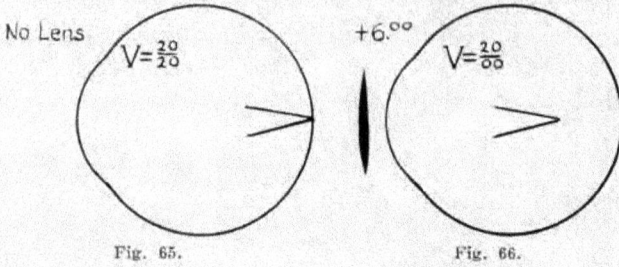

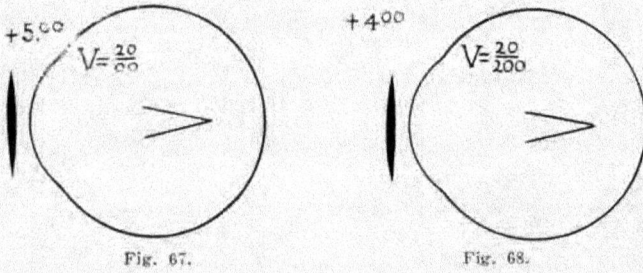

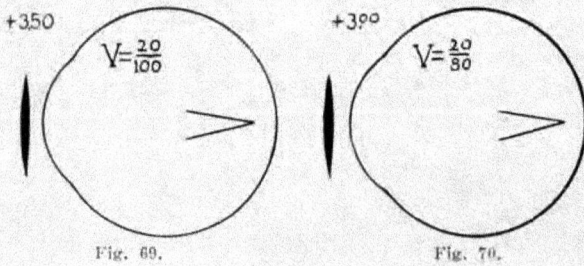

No Lens $V=\frac{20}{20}$

+6.⁰⁰ $V=\frac{20}{00}$

Fig. 65.　　　　Fig. 66.

+5.⁰⁰ $V=\frac{20}{00}$

+4⁰⁰ $V=\frac{20}{200}$

Fig. 67.　　　　Fig. 68.

+3.50 $V=\frac{20}{100}$

+3⁰⁰ $V=\frac{20}{80}$

Fig. 69.　　　　Fig. 70.

Experimental Correction of a Normal Eye.   (Emmetropia.)

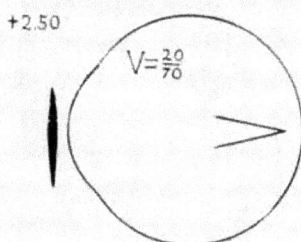

+2.50

$V=\frac{20}{70}$

Fig. 71

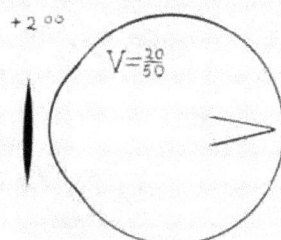

+2.00

$V=\frac{20}{50}$

Fig. 72

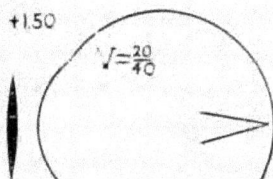

+1.50

$V=\frac{20}{40}$

Fig. 73

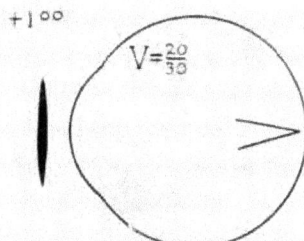

+1.00

$V=\frac{20}{30}$

Fig. 74

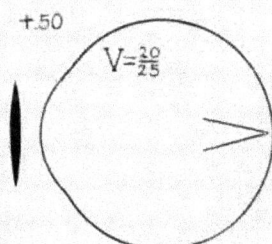

+.50

$V=\frac{20}{25}$

Fig. 75

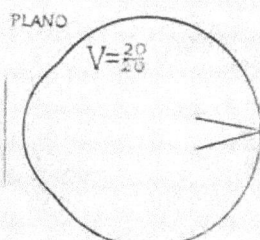

PLANO

$V=\frac{20}{20}$

Fig. 76

The Correction of Hypermetropia.

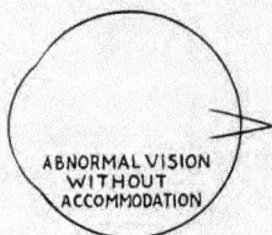

Fig. 77.

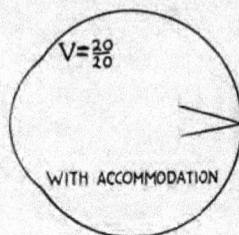

Fig. 78.

+ 6.

+ 5.50

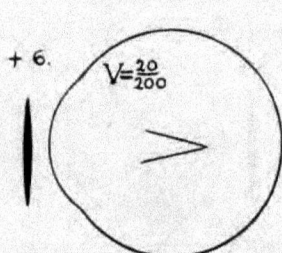

Fig. 79.

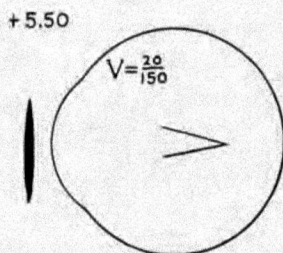

Fig. 80.

+ 5.

+ 4.50

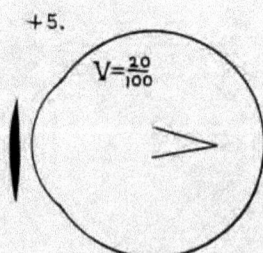

Fig. 81.

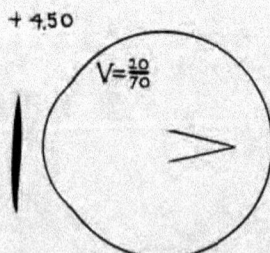

Fig. 82.

The Correction of Hypermetropia

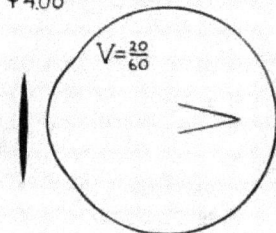

+4.00

$V = \frac{20}{60}$

Fig. 83

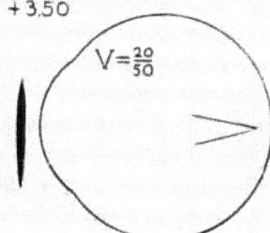

+3.50

$V = \frac{20}{50}$

Fig. 84

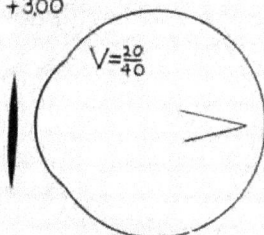

+3.00

$V = \frac{20}{40}$

Fig. 85

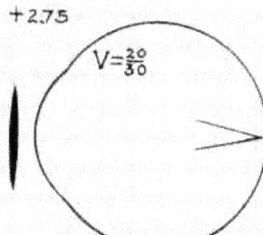

+2.75

$V = \frac{20}{30}$

Fig. 86

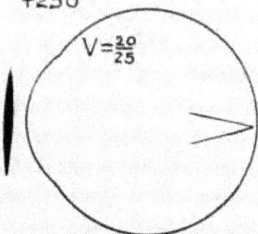

+2.50

$V = \frac{20}{25}$

Fig. 87

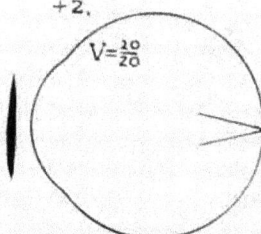

+2.

$V = \frac{20}{20}$

Fig. 88

The Correction of Myopia.

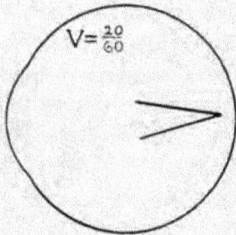

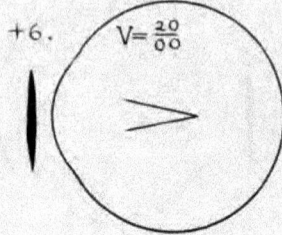

Fig. 89.   Fig. 90.

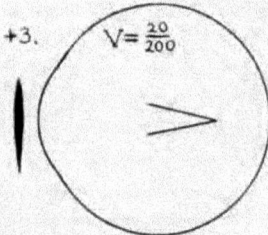

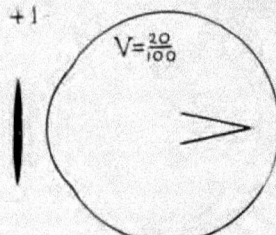

Fig. 91.   Fig. 92.

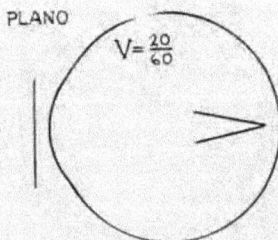

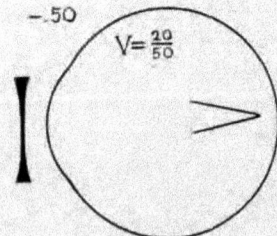

Fig. 93.   Fig. 94.

The Correction of Myopia

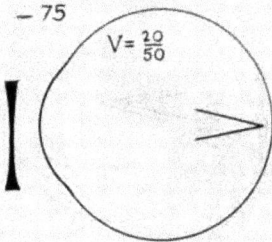

-75 $V = \dfrac{20}{50}$

Fig. 95

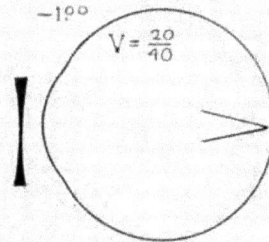

-1.00 $V = \dfrac{20}{40}$

Fig. 96

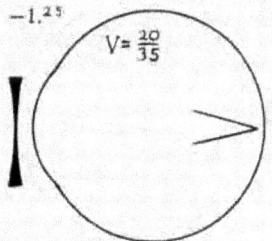

-1.25 $V = \dfrac{20}{35}$

Fig. 97

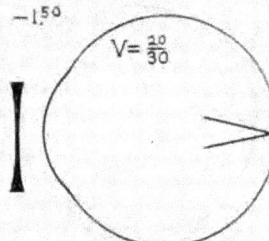

-1.50 $V = \dfrac{20}{30}$

Fig. 98

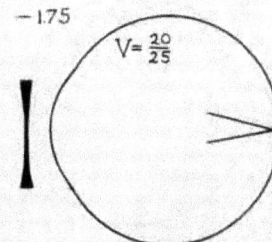

-1.75 $V = \dfrac{20}{25}$

Fig. 99

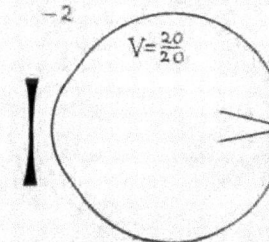

-2 $V = \dfrac{20}{20}$

Fig. 100

The Correction of Simple Myopic Astigmatism.

NO LENS
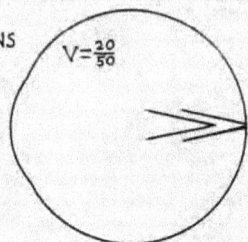

+6.
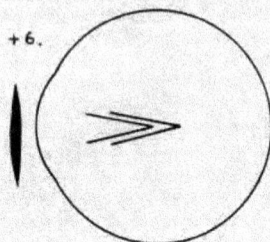

Fig. 101.

Fig. 102.

+5.
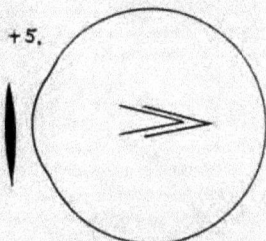

+4
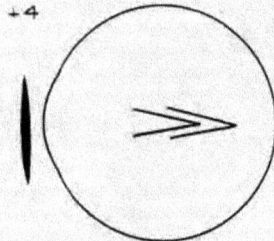

Fig. 103.

Fig. 104.

+3.
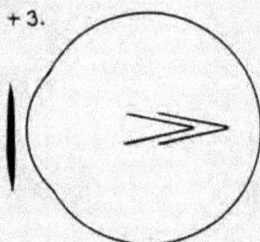

+2.
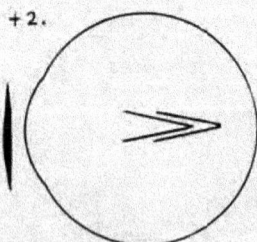

Fig. 105.

Fig. 106.

The Correction of Simple Myopic Astigmatism.

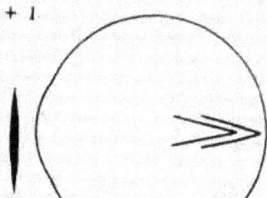
+ 1

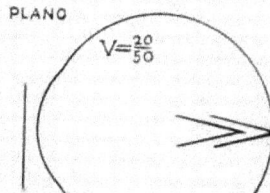
PLANO

$V=\frac{20}{50}$

Fig. 107   Fig. 108

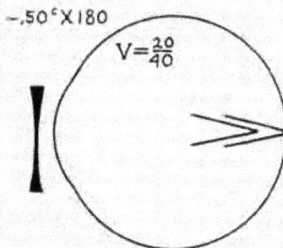
$-.50^c \times 180$

$V=\frac{20}{40}$

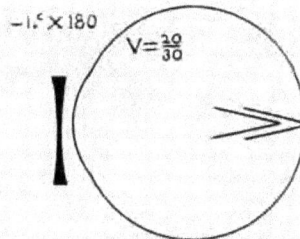
$-1.^c \times 180$

$V=\frac{20}{30}$

Fig. 109   Fig. 110

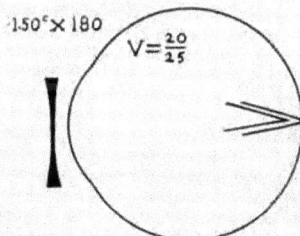
$-1.50^c \times 180$

$V=\frac{20}{25}$

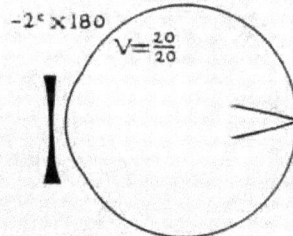
$-2^c \times 180$

$V=\frac{20}{20}$

Fig. 111   Fig. 112

The Correction of Simple Hypermetropic Astigmatism.

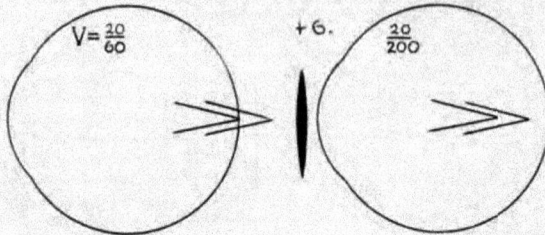

Fig. 113.   Fig. 114.

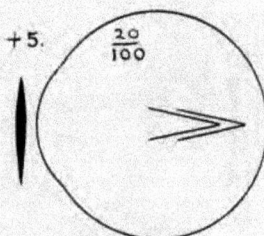

Fig. 115.

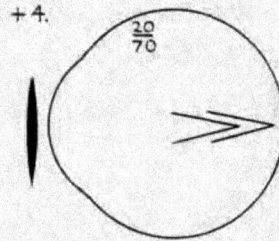

Fig. 116.

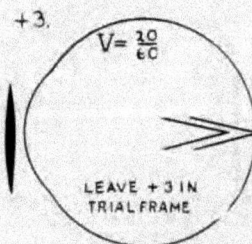

Fig. 117.

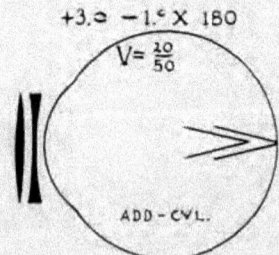

Fig. 118.

The Correction of Simple Hypermetropic Astigmatism.

+3.0 −1.50 ° X 180

$V = \frac{20}{40}$

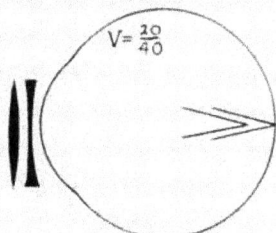

Fig. 119

+3.0 −2 ° X 180

$V = \frac{20}{35}$

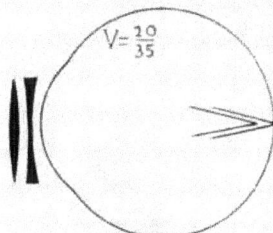

Fig. 120

+3.0 −2.50 ° X 180

$V = \frac{20}{30}$

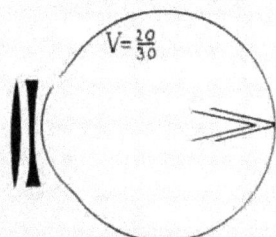

Fig. 121

+3.0 −2.75 ° X 180

$V = \frac{20}{20}$

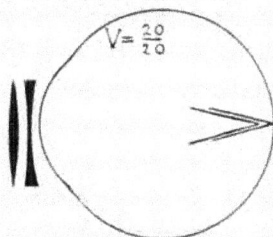

Fig. 122

+3.0 −3 ° X 180

$V = \frac{20}{15}$

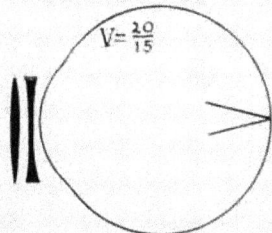

Fig. 123

+3. ° X 90

$V = \frac{20}{15}$

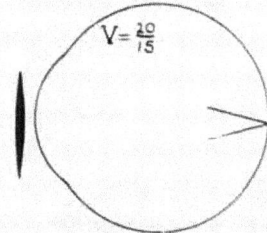

Fig. 124

The Correction of Compound Myopic Astigmatism.

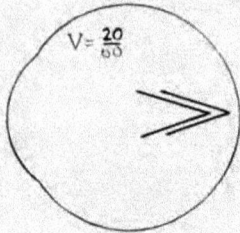
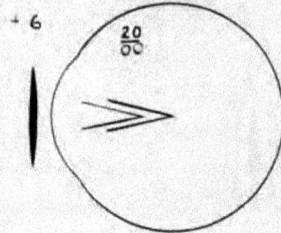

Fig. 125.   Fig. 126.

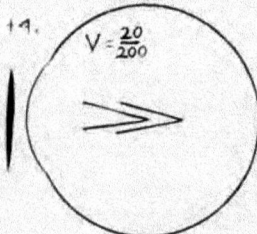
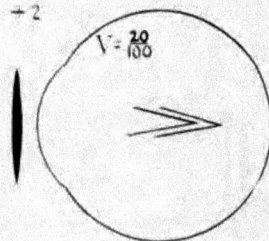

Fig. 127.   Fig. 128.

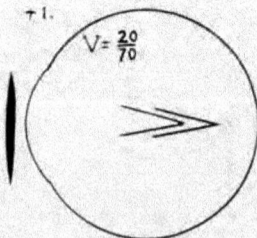
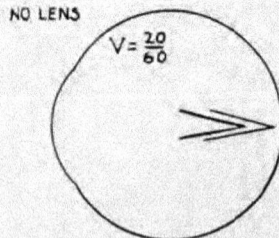

Fig. 129.   Fig. 130.

The Correction of Compound Myopic Astigmatism.

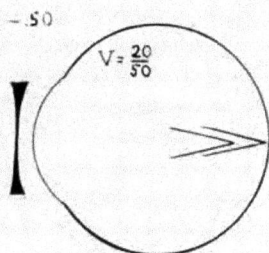

Fig. 131

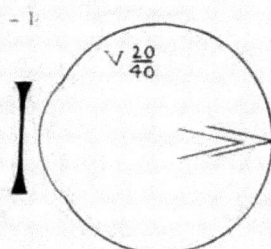

Fig. 132

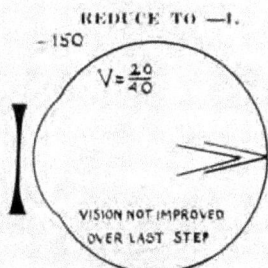

Fig. 133

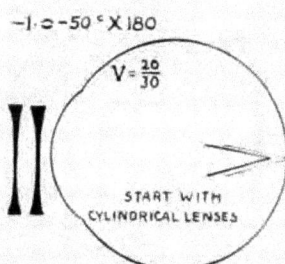

Fig. 134

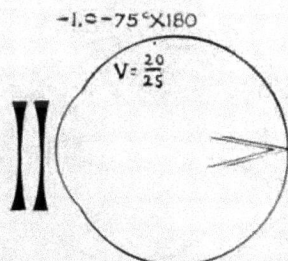

Fig. 135

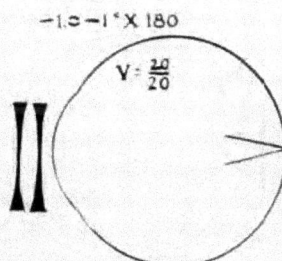

Fig. 136

The Correction of Compound Hypermetropic Astigmatism.

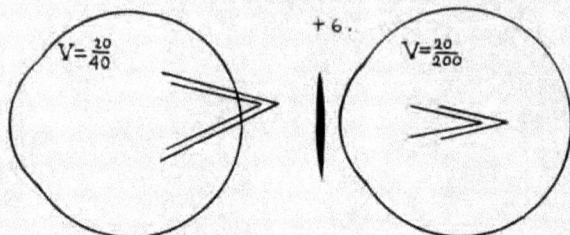

+6.

Fig. 137.   Fig. 138.

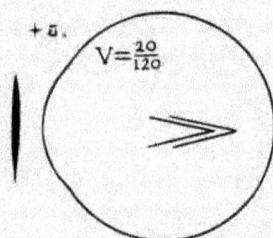
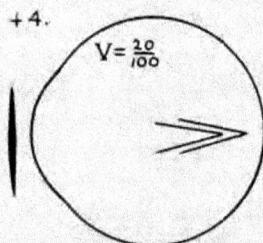

+5.   +4.

Fig. 139.   Fig. 140.

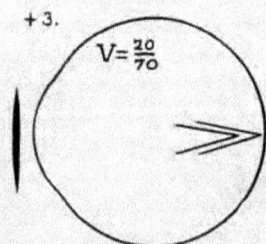
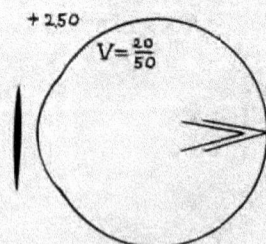

+3.   +2.50

Fig. 141.   Fig. 142.

The Correction of Compound Hypermetropic Astigmatism

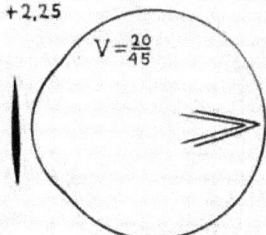

Fig. 143

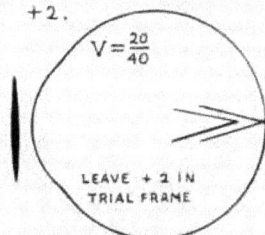

Fig. 144

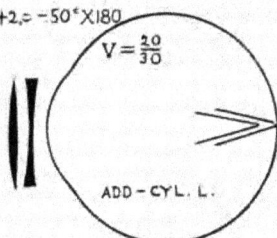

Fig. 145

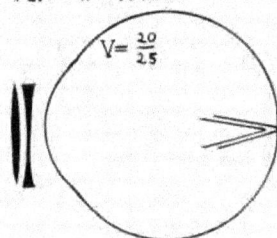

Fig. 146

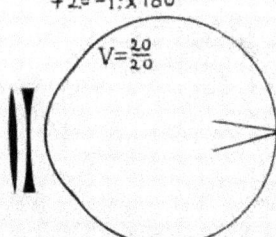

Fig. 147

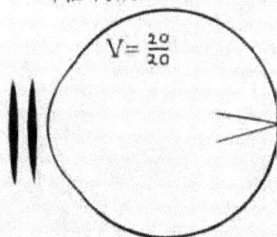

Fig. 148

The Correction of Mixed Astigmatism.

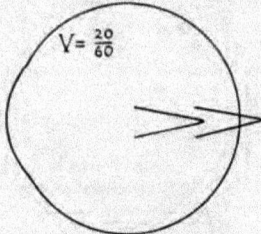

$V = \frac{20}{60}$

Fig. 149.

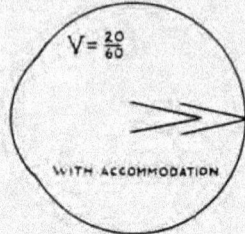

$V = \frac{20}{60}$

WITH ACCOMMODATION

Fig. 150.

+6.

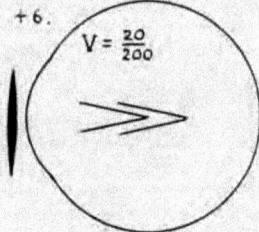

$V = \frac{20}{200}$

Fig. 151.

+5.

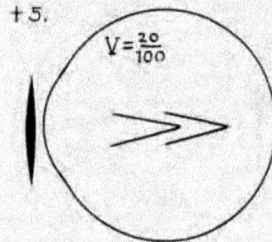

$V = \frac{20}{100}$

Fig. 152.

+3.

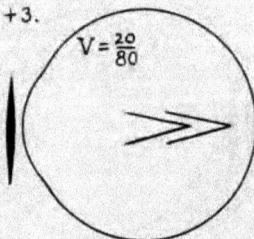

$V = \frac{20}{80}$

Fig. 153.

+1.50

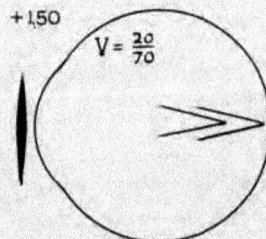

$V = \frac{20}{70}$

Fig. 154.

The Correction of Mixed Astigmatism.

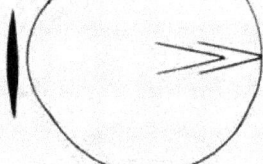
Fig. 155

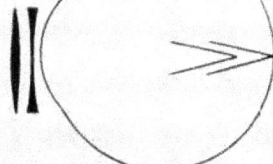
Fig. 156

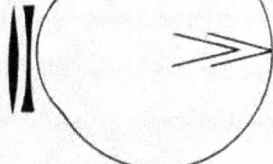
Fig. 157

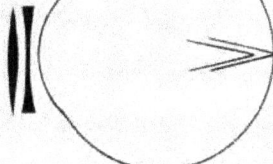
Fig. 158

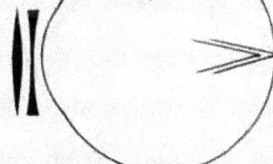
Fig. 159

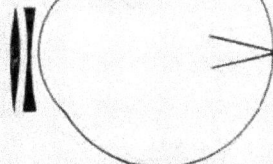
Fig. 160

Ingenious instruments have been devised to supplant the trial case for determining errors of refraction and are made without plus cylinders because they are unnecessary and superior claims are made both as to speed and accuracy by their makers. The instruments are constructed accurately and a descriptive pamphlet accompanies them.

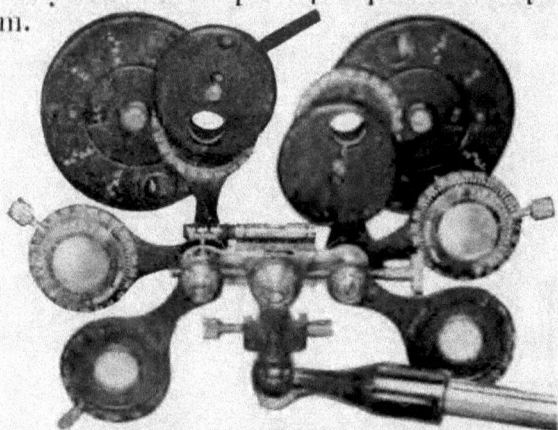

Fig. 161. Phoro-Optometer. (Hardy.)

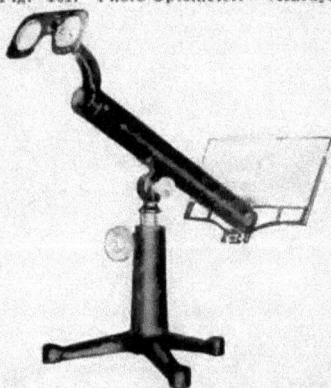

Fig. 162 Dynamic Refractor. (Hardy.)

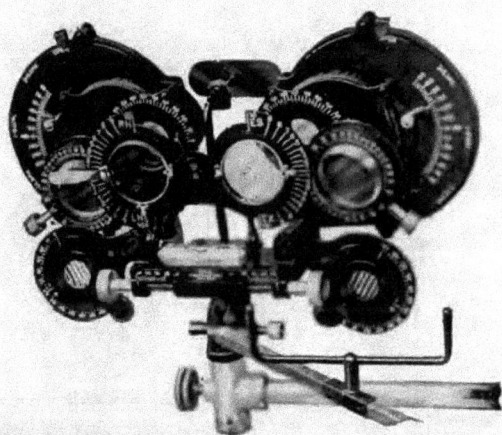

Fig. 163. Ski-Optometer. (Woolf.)

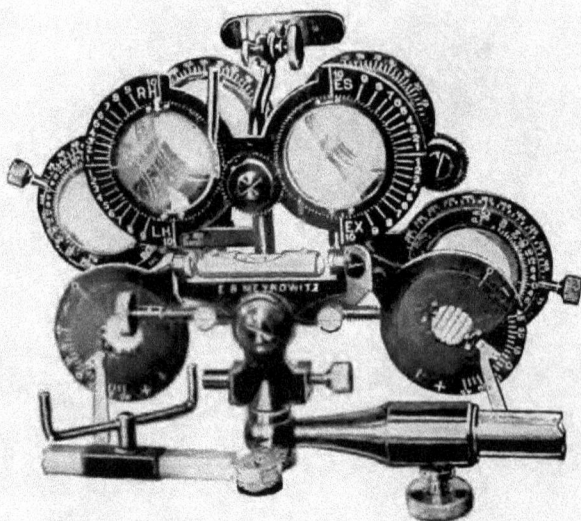

Fig. 164. Photometer Trial Frame. (Meyrowitz.)

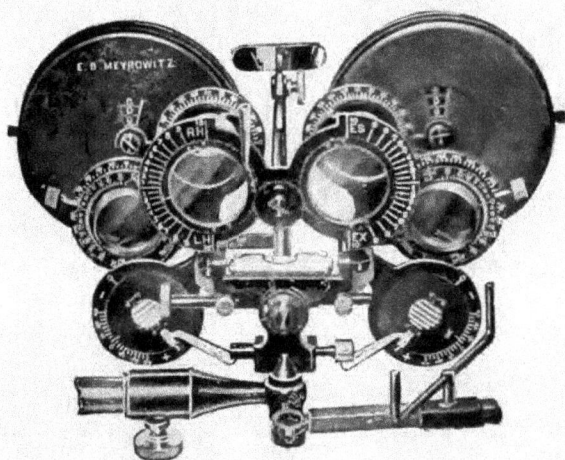

Fig. 165 Phoro-Optometer. (Meyerowitz.)

CYCLOPEGIA: The above rules apply when determining the manifest error as well as when examining for the static which must be preceded by putting the ciliary muscle at rest by the use of a cyclopegic.

HOMATROPIN: For transitory and incomplete cyclopegia we may use homatropin freshly prepared in 2% aqueous solution or in gelatin discs in the office for an hour immediately preceding refraction, making three instillations of the solution or applications of the discs at twenty minute intervals, and keeping the eyes bandaged during the intervening periods. Twenty minutes after the last instillation, the full effect of the drug will have been produced and the patient is ready for refraction. In adults, the cyclopegia thus produced is usually sufficient for this purpose.

ATROPIN: For a more complete and longer lasting cyclopegia, we usually make use of atropin sulphate in freshly prepared 1% aqueous solution for adults and ½% solution for children. The patient or nurse is given the solution, labeled poison, with instructions to instil one drop in each eye thrice daily for three days just prior to the refraction applying pressure to the lachrymal sacs for a moment after the instillation to prevent absorption from the nose and throat. Some operators use other cyclopegic alkaloids, but for most purposes, one or the other of the above will be found satisfactory.

SUGGESTION FOR THE USE OF CYCLOPEGICS:

Great care and adjustment is required in the use of cyclopegics, and while no positive rules can be laid down and each case must be considered on its own merits, the following suggestions as to their use will be found helpful:

1. All children under ten years of age should be refracted under cyclopegic. All cases of astigmatism should be corrected in full but some of the sphere should be deducted.

2. All cases of strabismus should be refracted likewise, and as full correction as will be tolerated prescribed.

3. Asthenopic patients who have not found relief with their manifest correction, should be similarly treated. All of the cylinder, and all of the manifest spherical, and part of the latent spherical is prescribed for constant wear.

4. If the manifest correction produces approximately normal vision in an asthenopic patient with subnormal vision, a cyclopegic will usually not be required.

5. Before using atropin in middle aged patients, carefully consider the possibility of producing glaucoma in that particular case.

6. Cyclopegics are rarely, if ever, required in patients over forty years of age and never in those over fifty.

CHAPTER IX

APPLIED REFRACTION

With these general considerations understood, we are ready to take up their application in the diagnosis and treatment of the refractive errors of the eyes, which, in this connection must be considered as most highly developed camerae obscurae functioning at once independently and in perfect unison. Considered optically, the normal eye may well be described as the ideal camera: having an iris diaphragm that acts automatically to meet the requirements of both illumination and focus as determined by the distance from the photographed object, a permanent sensitive plate and a method of focusing not by changing the length of the dark chamber; but by varying the dioptric strength of the refractive system from the static 43.5-D determined by dividing 100 centimeters by 23 millimeters, the length of the eye, required to focus images of objects beyond twenty feet to much more, making possible the focussing of the divergent rays given off by sources of illumination nearer than 20 feet. (Fig. 166.)

ACCOMMODATION: The function of thus increasing the dioptric strength of the lens system

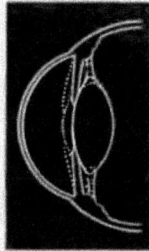

Fig. 166. Section of the Anterior Portion of the Eyeball. The dotted lines illustrate the changes during accommodation. (May.)

of the eye is called accommodation. The mechanism of its production is illustrated in Figure 166 showing how the action of the circular fibres of the ciliary muscle relaxes the suspensory ligament of the crystalline lens according to the theory of Helmholtz, the one usually accepted, which by its own elasticity increases its convexity; or according to the theory later advanced by Tscherning, who claims that in contraction the ciliary muscle compresses the suspensory ligament decreasing its circumference, thus similarly affecting the lens and forcing it to bulge in its antero-posterior diameter. However produced, the change in curvature takes place principally in the anterior surface, possibly because of the reduced resistance offered by the fluid aqueous as compared with that offered by the dense vitreous.

AMPLITUDE OF ACCOMMODATION: With the accommodation in abeyance, the crystalline lens exerts about 10 D. of the total (more than 40) possessed by the normal eye. But, as has been worked out by Donders, this amount is appreciably increased with the accommodation in force; the amount of increase, because of the gradual loss of lens elasticity with increasing years, varying inversely with the patient's age. The amount of possible increase of the accommodative function is called the amplitude of accommodation and is of very great importance in the consideration of hypermetropia and presbyopia, both of which will be discussed later. The results of Donder's work is set forth in the following table:

Amplitude of Accommodation

Age		Age	
10	14.00 D.	45	3.50 D.
15	12.00 D.	50	2.40 D.
20	10.00 D.	55	1.75 D.
25	8.50 D.	60	1.00 D.
30	7.00 D.	65	.75 D.
35	5.50 D.	70	.25 D.

With the optical principles of the previous chapter and the above dioptrics of the human eye well in mind, we will now take up the discussion of the diagnosis and treatment of refractive errors. Since it is the aim of this, as of all the chapters, to give the student a working, as well as an academic knowledge of the subjects discussed; and since all our cases come to us as unknown with the diagnosis to be worked out, we will endeavor to accomplish our aim by means of drawings.

CASE 1. J. S.—Bookkeeper, age 26, complains of irregular intermittent frontal headaches.

After preliminary ocular inspection with eversion and careful examination of the lids and palpation of the lacrymal sacs with negative results, he is comfortably seated at a distance of 20 feet from the well illumined Snellen chart, the trial frame properly adjusted, the left eye covered with the blank disc, and he is asked to read, when it is found that he can readily distinguish the letters in the line that should be read at 20 feet. A + .50 D. sphere is placed in the trial frame in front of his eye which blurs his vision perceptibly. The sphere is removed and a + .50 D. cylinder is placed before the eye with its axis at 90 and is immediately rejected as it is when turned to all other meridians. The patient is not hurried, the lenses are changed deftly and the questioning done tactfully and deliberately. While it is very unlikely that the eye can be myopic with normal vision, a minus .50 sphere is now inserted and the patient reports on questioning that the lens seems to put a strain on the eye although he can see as well or perhaps a little better with it than without. Accordingly, the sphere is removed and a — .50 D. cylinder inserted with its axis at 180 with a similar result which continues when its axis is slowly rotated through an arc of 90°. The lens is removed and the blank disc taken from the left eye and placed over the right and the former refracted as was the right and with a similar result.

It is decided that the patient has no manifest error. In order to be absolutely certain, the patient was asked to return next day for examination under a cyclopegic, when after the use of homatropin as previously described and after a repetition of the above procedures, the same results were verified by retinoscopy. (See Chapter XI.)

We are therefore forced to the conclusion that the refractive condition of his eyes is normal and that the cause of the headaches must be sought for in some other condition of the eyes or even in some other structure, if during the remainder of the complete systematic ocular examination, no condition is found warranting the symptoms complained of.

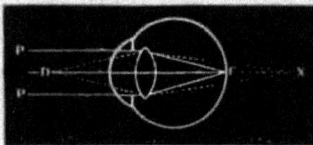

Fig. 167. The Emmetropic Eye in a State of Rest. (May.)   Fig. 168. The Emmetropic Eye During Accommodation. (May.)

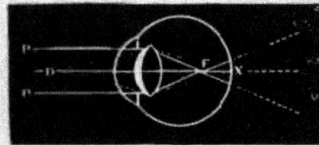

EMMETROPIA: Emmetropia (Figure 167) is that condition in which with the accommodation in abeyance, the relation of dioptric strength to the antero-posterior diameter of the eye is such that all rays of light originating beyond 20 feet from the eye are brought to a focus on the retina. In other words, the eye may be said to be at rest when looking at a distance thus saving all of the accommodative force for near work as shown in Figure 168.

As mentioned above, people with normal eyes frequently come to us seeking relief from symptoms which they erroneously attribute to eye conditions and we must be able to diagnose emmetropia as accurately as we do ametropia. Indeed we must know the normal if we are to recognize a deviation from it. In the above case the wearing of any lenses other than absolutely neutral ones would be undesirable.

In an earlier chapter, we emphasized the importance of making ocular examinations systematically. The author wishes to reiterate that statement here, to emphasize the importance in the use of the trial case, and to describe and illustrate a system for its use which being faithfully followed will give the nearest possible accuracy of results.

Case II. Miss A. C.—Stenographer, Aged 22. Complains that eyes tire quickly at her work and that severe occipital headaches come on during the afternoon. She is wearing + 0.75 D. each eye.

Following the rules for refraction, pages 132-163, we arrive at the following result:

R. E. 20/15 + 1.25 = 20/15.

L. E. 20/15 + 1.50 = 20/15.

The diagnosis of the above and of the following four cases of hypermetropia with its correction by lenses is shown in the following figures.

HYPERMETROPIA: In hypermetropia, there is a disturbance in the relation between dioptric power and length of eye as a result of which, with the accommodation in abeyance, parallel rays of light reach the retina having come to a focus as is shown in Figure 169.

While the condition is usually thought of as the result of shortening of the antero-posterior diameter as shown in Figure 170, it may be caused by a deficiency of the static refraction of the eye by exertion of the accommodative function.

If the deficiency is within amplitude of accommodation, the patient may be able to maintain clear distant vision more or less constantly, with usually a more or less complete failure of the function for near work

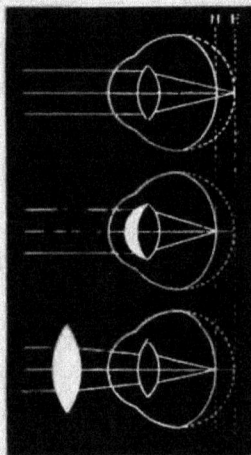

Fig. 169. Hypermetropic Eye in a State of Rest. (May.)
Fig. 170. Hypermetropic Eye During Accommodation. (May.)
Fig. 171. Hypermetropia Corrected by a Convex Lens. (May.)

and some or all of the symptoms of eye strain. How this same end may be served by a convex lens, giving constant clear, easy, distant vision and conservation of the accommodative function for its normal use in near vision is shown in Figure 171.

CASE III. R. R., Aged 35. Laborer. Complains of recent failure of distant vision. States

that he never was able to read for any length of
time. The rules on page 132 were followed with
result as follows:

R. E. 20/50 + 4.50 sph. = 20/20

L. E. 20/60 + 5.00 sph. = 20/20.

Given above for constant wear.

CASE IV. Master G. L., Aged 5. Mother
states that left eye has turned in for last three
or more years. The manifest was taken according to the rules, page 132 using the illiterate
chart.

R. E. 20/40 + 2.50 = 20/20

L. E. 20/80 + 4.00 = 20/50

The mother was given a ½% aqueous solution
of atropin sulphate with instructions to instil
two drops in each eye morning, noon, and night,
and requested to bring the child in three days
when the following results verified by the use of
the retinoscope were obtained.

R. E. 20/100 + 4.00 = 20/20

L. E. 20/200 + 5.50 = 20/50

Given right eye + 3.50 sph. — left eye + 5.00
sph. with instructions to use one drop of ½%
solution of atropin sulphate in each eye before
retiring every third day and to report at the end
of one month for examination.

CASE V. Miss M. H., Age 25. Teacher.
Complains that glasses she is now wearing which
were fitted two months ago have failed to relieve
frontal headache and epiphora complained of at
that time.

R. E. 20/20 + .50 = 20/20

L. E. 20/20 + .50 = 20/20

Examination of her glasses show them to be the same. Three instillations of a 2% solution of homatropin hydrobromate were made at twenty minute intervals and the refraction repeated twenty minutes after the last instillation with the following results:

R. E. 20/40 + 1.75 sph. = 20/20
L. E. 20/40 + 1.75 sph. = 20/20

Given plus 1.00 sph. both eyes with instructions to use them constantly and to report the result in a week.

CASE VI. N. A., Aged 23. Electrician. States that while taking a civil service examination recently it was discovered that he did not have useful vision in his left eye. Following the rules page 132 in order we find the following:

R. E. 20/20 + .50 = 20/15
L. E. 20/200 + 4.50 = 20/30

In practice it is found that a difference of more than about four dioptres will not be accepted because the difference in size of the retinal images makes binocular vision impossible. Since he complains of no discomfort nor other symptoms he was advised not to wear glasses.

CASE VII. Miss J. C., Aged 40. Bookkeeper. Comes wearing glasses which she states she had been advised to wear to save her eyes and which have always been uncomfortable although according to the rules we find first that the visual acuity is 20/30 in the right eye and that neither convex spheres nor cylinders improve it. Concave spheres are found to help a — .75 D. sphere giving a visual acuity of 20/20 which is not im-

proved by a concave cylinder. A similar result
was obtained with the left eye so we have:

R. E. 20/30 — .75 sph. = 20/20

L. E. 20/30 — .75 sph. = 20/20

She was asked to return for examination under
cyclopegia which done the next day gave the following:

R. E. 20/40 — .50 = 20/20

L. E. 20/40 — .50 = 20/20

She was advised not to wear glasses as in her
refractive condition there was no inconvenience
other than a slight impairment of distant vision.
so slight as to be disregarded. In this as in the

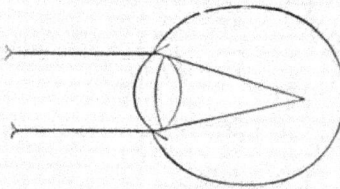

Fig. 172. Myopic Eye. (Thoring-   Fig. 173. Myopic Eye Corrected by
ton.)   Concave Lens. (Thorington.)

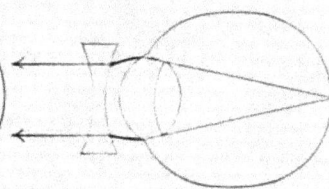

following two cases the refractive error is called
Myopia. This is described as a disturbance of
the relation between dioptric power and length
of eye; and is the opposite of that in hypermetropia, that is, with the eye at rest. parallel rays are
focussed within the eye and crossing produces a
circle of diffusion on the retina with resultant
poor distant vision as shown in figure 172.

While the condition may be due to excessive
static refraction. it is usually caused by actual
increase of the antero-posterior diameter of the

eye. Figure 173 shows the same eye with the proper concave lens before it which causes the parallel rays to diverge just enough to have them focus on the retina after having passed through the eye's dioptric system with the accommodation at rest.

CASE VIII. H. H. Aged 12—Student.

Referred by teacher who has observed that distant vision is subnormal as evidenced by inability to see work on blackboard from rear of room. Applying rules page 132 one to five in order, we have:

R. E. 20/80 — 2.50 sph. = 20/25
L. E. 20/100 — 3.00 sph. = 20/25

Which correction when tried for a few moments in the office was found to tire the eyes for near work and the following correction, with which near work would be comfortably done, was given for constant wear.

R. E. — 1.50 sph. = 20/40
L. E. — 2.00 sph. = 20/40

The strongest glass a myopic patient can read with comfort, will usually be worn with satisfaction.

CASE IX. Miss J. B. Aged 30—Seamstress.

Complains of inability to see at distance without strong minus glasses.

R. E. 20/200 — 6.00 sph. = 20/40
L. E. 20/100 — 5.00 sph. = 20/30

This correction gave satisfactory distant vision but could not be used for near work.

R. E. — 3.00 sph. distant vision 20/60
L. E. — 2.00 sph. distant vision 20/50

Since this gave too poor distant vision to be of use, she was given two pair of glasses which proved quite satisfactory. Full correction for distant and for work R. — 3.00 sph. L. — 2.00 sph.

CAUSES OF ASTIGMATISM: An equal refraction in different meridians of the same eye may be due either to an irregularity of the cornea or of the lens, but practically is the result of combined conditions in both of them as is shown by the fact that often eyes having a moderate corneal astig-

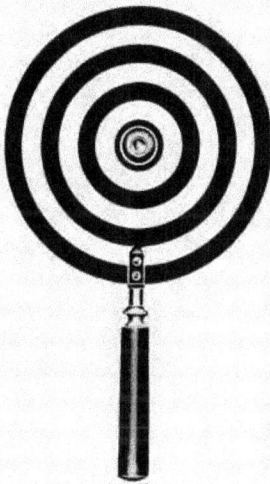

Fig 175   Corneal Reflection of Placedo's Disc in Emmetropia.

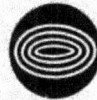

Fig. 176.   Corneal Reflection of Placedo's Disc in Regular Astigmatism.

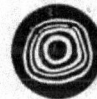

Fig. 174.   Keratoscope

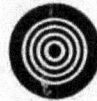

Fig. 177.   Corneal Reflection of Placedo's Disc in Irregular Astigmatism. (May.)

matism are free from the condition when the entire dioptric apparatus is considered— the corneal astigmatism is corrected by a lenticular one.

MEANS OF DIAGNOSIS OF ASTIGMATISM: In addition to the subjective methods to be described for determining and measuring the amount of the condition, we have certain objective ones for diagnosing it. One of the earliest devised instruments for use in this connection is Placedo's keratoscope. (Figure 174.)

Consists of a disc on the face of which are painted alternating concentric black and white circles to which is attached a handle for convenience in handling. When this disc is held before

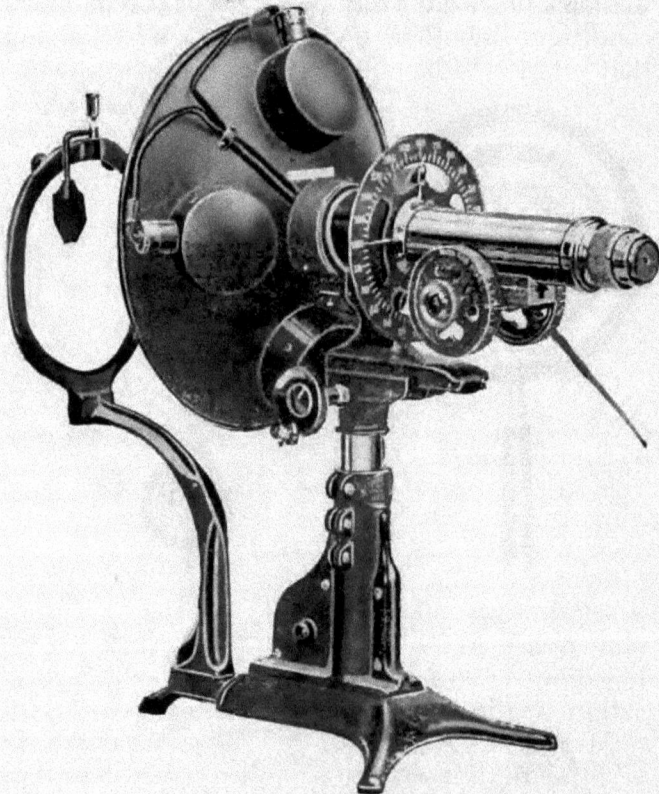

Fig 178. Ophthalmometer. (Hardy.)

an eye its reflection assumes one of the forms
illustrated. (Figs. 175, 176 and 177.)

Another instrument for investigating the corneal curvatures is the ophthalmometer, Figure
178, directions for the use of which accompany
the instrument.

The student will note that both of the above
instruments investigate the condition of the cornea only, and he will bear in mind that the corneal error may be corrected by the proper defect
in the lens. There is one means, however, of
gaining information concerning the total condition resulting from both corneal and lenticular
irregularity, and that is by the application of
direct ophthalmoscopy. If, on looking at the
disc, it is observed to be distinctly oval, there is
a very great likelihood of the eye being astigmatic; and, if the refraction of the eye by means
of this instrument, as shown by refracting the
vessels running at right angles to each other, is
different in different meridians, the condition is
positively diagnosed.

FORMS OF ASTIGMATISM: Astigmatism or
curvature ametropia is described as regular when
there is no break in the continuity of any of the
refracting surfaces, and the difference in their
curvature proceeds regularly from that of minimum radius to that of the minimum one when the
keratascope produces an image similar to the one
illustrated in Figure 176.

When there is a break in the surface of any of
the refracting mediae or their curvatures do not
proceed regularly as described above, an irregu-

lar astigmatism is produced which is not correctible with lenses. Practically this can occur with the cornea only as the result of injury or disease and the keratascope image will resemble that shown in Figure 177.

The condition is further described as "with the rule" when the eye's greatest dioptric power lies in or near the vertical meridians, the usual condition, and which is attributed to shortening of the radius of curvature of the cornea by lid pressure. When the greatest dioptric power lies in or near the horizontal meridian the astigmatism is described as "against the rule."

REGULAR ASTIGMATISM: These are also considered as forms of the basic ametropias and in this connection are described as compound Hyperopic astigmatism of which the last case is an example.

1. Simple Hyperopic Astigmatism (Page 181), in which the eye is hypermetropic in one meridian and is emmetropic in the one at right angles to it.

2. Simple Myopic Astigmatism (Page 181), in which one meridian is emmetropic and the other myopic.

3. Compound Hypermetropic Astigmatism, (Page 181) in which both meridians are hypermetropic, but to a different degree.

4. Compound Myopic Astigmatism, (Page 181) in which both meridians are myopic but to a different degree.

5. Mixed Astigmatism (Page 181), where

one meridian is hypermetropic and the other myopic.

All of the above five forms may be either with or against the rule and are correctible with lenses.

SYMPTOMS OF ASTIGMATISM: If the astigmatic error be high in amount, the only symptom usually noted is a low visual acuity; but, if it exists in only a moderate degree and the patient has an active accommodation, he may suffer with the most marked asthenopic symptoms especially if engaged in work calling for accurate vision because of the eye's efforts to produce it by constant varying of the amount of ciliary muscle action in use. Any or all of the symptoms that are complained of may be described and all usually disappear promptly with the wearing of the proper correcting lenses.

PREVALENCE AND IMPORTANCE OF ASTIGMATISM: Curvature ametropia with its many forms is the most common of refractive troubles, and considered on the basis of the discomfort it causes, it is undoubtedly the most important. Likewise, it is the most difficult to estimate accurately which has resulted in the development of numerous accessory devices and various special charts for use in subjective refracting. Of the accessories, all may well be discarded save the stenopic slit, which will often be found useful in locating the principal meridians when they have not been located by other methods.

STENOPIC SLIT: Figure 53. This accessory is used by placing it in the properly adjusted trial frame and asking the patient to look at the Snellen chart, the operator meanwhile rotating the cell of the trial frame.

If the patient sees better in one meridian than in others, very likely he is astigmatic, and the meridian at which he sees best, which should be accepted only after several revolutions of the disc preferably by the patient himself, is one of the principal meridians. In this event, he will have the poorest vision while using the slit when it is rotated to ninety degrees from the first one chosen. Some operators use the stenopic slit throughout the work with the trial case refracting each meridian separately, and combining the results for the prescription, but this is not to be recommended.

ASTIGMATIC CHARTS: Numerous special astigmatic charts, all modifications of the clock dial chart (Figure 61), have been devised, but they are not to be recommended since they really are little or no improvement over the original without which some operators get along very well depending on visual results alone as determined with the Snellen type.

Case X. C. J. Aged 25—Telegrapher.

Complains of frontal headaches that increase toward evening. On refracting systematically we find:

R. E. 20/20 + .50 cyl. ax. 90 = 20/20.

L. E. 20/20 + .37 cyl. ax. 90 = 20/20.

Under homatropin the following was secured:

R. E. 20/60 + .75 sph. ⌐ + .50 cyl. ax. 90 = 20/20.

L. E. 20 60 + .75 sph. ‏⸮‎ + .37 cyl. ax. 90 = 20 20.

He was given:

R. E. + .25 sph. ‏⸮‎ + .50 cyl. ax. 90.

L. E. + .25 sph. ‏⸮‎ + .37 cyl. ax. 90.

DIAGNOSIS: Compound Hypermetropic Astigmatism. Figure 133.

CASE XI. J. J. Aged 22—Porter.

Complains of poor distant and near vision. With the regular procedure we find the vision R. E. to be 20 80 plus spheres are rejected but plus cylinders with the axis at 135 are accepted readily as they are in the left eye, save that the axis is at 45. The result is as follows:

R. E. 20 80 P. H. 20 30 + 2.50 ax. 135 20 30.

L. E. 20 100 P. H. 20 40 + 3.00 ax. 45 20 40.

DIAGNOSIS: Simple Hypermetropic Astigmatism. Figure 179.

CASE XII. Mrs. G. F. Age 23—Housewife.

Complains of poor vision, epiphora and headaches. Applying the rules in order we find:

R. E. 20 80 + 1.25 cyl. ax. 100 = 20 50 ‏⸮‎ — .75 cyl. ax. 10 = 20 20.

L. E. 20 65 + 1.00 cyl. ax. 100 = 20 40 ‏⸮‎ — .50 cyl. ax. 10 = 20 20.

DIAGNOSIS: Mixed Astigmatism.

CASE XIII. A. C. Aged 35—Bookkeeper.

Complains of usual symptoms for near work and states that condition has been increasing since beginning to wear present correction ten days ago. Examining systematically, we find that plus spheres and cylinders are rejected and that a —.50 sphere improves the vision. R. E. from 20. 60 to 20/40 and that a —.50 D. cylinder improves anywhere near 180 degrees. Using the stenopic slit, we determine the location of the meridian as at 170 degrees and apply one cylinder with axis at that point.

Completing the refraction of that and the left eye we have:

R. E. 20/60 P. H. 20/30 — .50 sph. ◯ — .75 cyl. ax. 170 = 20/20.

L. E. 20/80 P. H. 20/30 — .75 sph. ◯ — 1.00 cyl. ax. 10 = 20/25.

DIAGNOSIS: Compound myopic astigmatism. Figure 179.

Examination of his glasses found him to be wearing the same lenses save that the axes were at 180 degrees. They were given to him with the axis at the proper position with very satisfactory results.

APHAKIA: There remains one more anomaly of the static refraction of the eye, a high degree of hypermetropia or more often compound hypermetropic astigmatism, produced artificially either by complete dislocation of the crystalline lens within the vitreous, or more often by its removal because of its being cataractous. After such dislocation or removal, the eye is said to be aphakic.

THE CORRECTION OF APHAKIA: In the correction of this condition, the same rules are followed, but practice has demonstrated that roughly speaking a + 10 D. sphere will be required to take the place of the removed lens with or without a cylinder to correct the corneal deformity resulting from the incision. Another practical point is that when using the pin hole disc to determine the visual acuity that may be expected—that the placing a + 10 D. sphere before it in the trial frame usually give better results.

Since the cylinder, if required at all, is usually of considerable strength, great care must be exercised in locating its axis correctly. The use of the stenopic slit will prove of very great assistance in doing this. Often the distortion of the test chart with a + 5 D. sphere before the eye will give a valuable clue to the location of the axis.

Since changes in the dioptric power of the eye continue for some little time after the operation. an aphakic patient should not have his correction prescribed until six weeks have elapsed after his discharge; one other thing that must be remembered is that a monocular aphakic patient cannot wear his correction if he has normal or nearly normal vision in his other eye. However, he should be refracted so that you and he may know just what vision he may expect in the event of the other eye becoming incapacitated.

CASE XIV. L. A. Aged 24. Laborer. Swollen opaque lens resulting from penetrating injury ten days previously, removed from right eye eight weeks ago because of secondary glaucoma, applying the rules we have.

R. E. 20/200 P. H. + 10.00 = 20/20 + 6.00
 + 2.00 ax. 80 = 20/20.
 L. E. 20/20 + .25 = 20/20.
Glasses were not prescribed because they would
not be practical.

CASE XV. J. C. Aged 69. Farmer. Both
lenses removed six weeks ago because of senile
cataract. Following the rules:

R. E. 10/200 P. H. 20/25 + 9.00 = 20/25.
 L. E. 15/200 + 8.00 + 1 cyl. ax. 105 = 20/25
P. H. 20/25.

Given above for distance with suitable correction for reading as discussed under presbyopia.

RECAPITULATION: This completes the discussion of the static errors of refraction which will
be closed by again emphasizing the need of following the rules page 142 or pages 138-153 in
the order given and which are epitomized in the
following combined figure and table.

In the normal eye a + 50 sph or cyl would diminish the visual acuity, so would — sph and — cyl lenses. Any of them would remove the focal point from the retina.

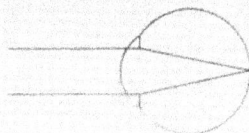

In hyperopia, a + 50 sph would improve vision, rays of light being converged and brought forward on the retina.

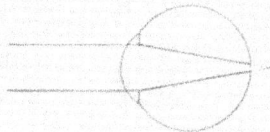

In comp. hyperopic astigmatism, a + sph lens will improve the vision and combining a + cyl lens with it would correct the defect.

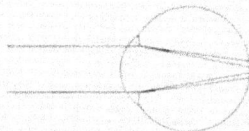

In simple hyperopic astigmatism, a + sph would not improve vision; a + cyl lens would converge rays of light in one median, bringing it on the retina.

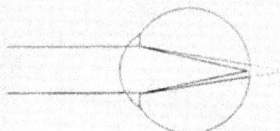

In mixed astigmatism, + sph or — sph lenses will not improve the error. A + cyl lens would improve it and a — cyl lens at right angles in the former would correct the error.

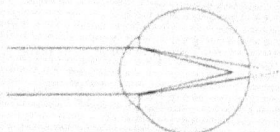

In myopic astigmatism, a + sph would not improve vision; a — cyl lens with the sph would correct the error.

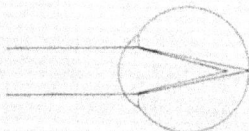

In myopia a +50 sph or + 50 cyl would decrease the vision; a — sph would diverge the rays of light and bring the focus on the retina.

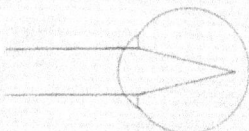

In comp. myopic astigmatism a — sph lens would improve the vision; a — cyl lens with the sph would correct the error.

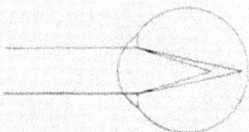

Fig. 179.

PRESBYOPIA: In an earlier section, the function of accommodation was considered and mention made of the fact of its gradual failure from youth to age with an accompanying table giving its amplitude at various ages. The individual is unconscious of this gradual loss of accommodative power until it becomes so reduced as to make near work difficult or even impossible.

Since the great portion of near work is done at about 13 inches, the equivalent of approximately a + 3.50 D. sphere must be maintained to focus the divergent rays originating from this nearby source of illumination on the retina of the emmetropic eye whether it occur naturally or be by lenses.

ONSET OF PRESBYOPIA: A glance at the table referred to will show that the eye usually has just this amount of accommodative power at the forty-fifth year and that it is gradually reduced until it is practically absent at the seventieth year. Forty-five then is said to be the age of the onset of presbyopia because it is at that time that the need for assisting the failing accommodation with stronger and stronger convex spheres begins.

AMOUNT OF ADDITION REQUIRED: In determining the strength of the convex spheres added, the eye must always be considered as emmetropic. If hypermetropic, the static correction must be added to that given for age, and, if myopic, must be deducted from it.

Incidently, it should be noted that the onset of presbyopia is hastened by uncorrected hypermetropia; that it is delayed by myopia. It is not

nature's plan to ever make use of the entire quantity of any force but rather to hold some little of
it in reserve for emergencies. For this reason it
is found advisable to supply a little more plus, as
we say, than is actually required for the usual
working distance. This gives the eye a small reserve for occasional near work and makes possible a greater delicacy of adjustment for fine
work. The following table gives the strength
of the convex lens usually required at different
ages, but must not be followed exactly because
of the individual variations in the onset of degree of presbyopia and the varying working distance of people of different occupations.

TABLE FOR PRESBYOPIC
CORRECTION

Age	Addition required.
45	1. D. Sphere.
50	2. D. Sphere.
55	2.50 Sphere.
60	3.00 Sphere.

Presbyopic correction of Aphakic Patients:
Since the aphakic patient obviously has no accommodation whatever, he may quite properly
be regarded as an individual of seventy-five years
in so far as his eyes are concerned, and be given
the full amount of near correction required for
the working distance decided upon, usually three-
and-one-half dioptres.

NEAR TEST TYPE: The numbering of the Jaeger type described in the previous chapter has been changed in recent years so that noting the finest type the patient can read when made emmetropic, the variously sized sections are captioned with strength of the plus sphere that likely will be required to give him normal near vision. The chart like the table must be considered and treated individually, seeking to give the clearest near vision with the greatest range possible.

ILLUSTRATED CASES: Case XVIII—Mrs. J. T., Aged 41. Housewife.

Complains that eyes tire at near work for last three months; has never worn glasses and has recently been through a severe illness.

EXAMINATION shows her to be emmetropic but unable to read the finest type which is made clear over a wide range with a + .50 D. sphere before both eyes.

Given above for near work only.

CASE XV. E. B., Aged 50. Farmer.

Complains of inability to read comfortably for last month. Found to be hypermetropic one-half dioptre in both eyes and to require the addition of a + .75 D. sphere before both eyes to make the finest type clear. Given:

R. E. + 1.25 |
L. E. + 1.25 | for near work.

CHAPTER X

HETEROPHORIA—MUSCULAR INSUFFICIENCY

Orthorphoria: Perfect binocular balance.

Heterophoria: Imperfect binocular balance.

Esophoria: A tendency of the visual axis inward.

Hyperesophoria: A tendency of the visual axis upward and inward.

Exophoria: A tendency of the visual axis of one eye to turn out.

Hyperexophoria: A tendency of the visual axis of one eye to be above the other and outward.

Hypophoria: A tendency of the axis of one eye to be below the other.

Squint: Cross eye, or an actual deviation of one of the eyes in, out, up or down.

Much has been written and very little is understood about extrinsic ocular muscle anomalies. Many theories have been advanced for the occurrence and correction of the heterophoria; but the fact remains that they often disappear spontaneously on wearing the refractive correction and that they seldom yield to treatment by means of prism exercises, which however, should be tried before resorting to operative procedures.

DIAGNOSIS OF MUSCULAR ERRORS: Tests for muscular anomalies should always be made with the patient wearing the refractive correction since very often there is much less insufficiency with the lenses than there is when they are not worn. The tests all depend on placing the muscular fusion sense in abeyance which is accomplished by making the images in the two eyes so different as to make these fusions into one impossible.

Various accessories have been developed for this purpose but none are better than the Maddox Rod before one eye and a colored disc before the other when the patient is instructed to look at a small light at a distance in a moderately darkened room. Under these conditions, the eye wearing the Maddox Rod sees a streak of light at right angles to the direction of the rod; and the other one, of course, sees a colored light. If they coincide the eyes are in a state of muscular balance; if not, the strength of prism placed with bases over the weaker muscles required to make the images coincide is the measure of the heterophoria. Either the horizontal or vertical muscles may be tested by simply rotating the rod, thus changing the direction of the streak.

In addition to determining the static condition by the above method, one should always determine the measure of the muscular action with the fusion sense acting. This is done by having the patient look at the light while wearing his correction and determining the strength of the prism with which he can maintain single vision. Remember that the apex must be placed over the muscle tested. The normal individual should overcome from one to two prism dioptres base up or down; four to six, base in; and from twelve to eighteen base out.

PRISM TREATMENT OF HETEROPHORIA: When a heterophoria does not disappear on wearing the correction, efforts should be made to develop the deficient pair of muscles by means of appropriate prism exercises. In using prisms to exercise muscles, one must remember to place the apex of the lens over the muscle to be exercised and to attempt to so gauge the length and frequency of treatment and increase of prism as to stimulate the muscle rather than to fatigue it.

OPERATIVE TREATMENT OF HETEROPHORIA: Exophoria, or a deviation of the axis outward is the usual muscle imbalance requiring operative treatment, the technique of which is the same as operations for squint or cross eyes, and the author believes a tenotomy of the external rectus with a retaining suture should be done, but not until an attempt to correct the refractive error has been made.

CHAPTER X

RETINOSCOPY

Retinoscopy is a method of estimating the refraction of the eye by studying the movements and form of the retinal reflex obtained by throwing a beam of light from a plane mirror into the eye from a given distance.

APPARATUS

The apparatus necessary for this work is a plane retinoscopic mirror of about one and one-half inches in diameter, a good light, (preferably on an adjustable bracket), trial frame and case of trial lenses. As to the light, an Argand gas burner or an electric lamp, spherical in shape and frosted to prevent an image of the filament showing, are the best, although a good clear candle or oil lamp will do.

The best place in which to do retinoscopy is an absolutely dark room, but an outside room with the windows shaded by opaque shades answers all purposes.

SCHEMATIC EYE

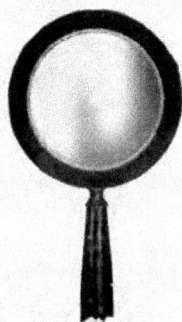

For study by the beginner, the best device is a good schematic eye (Figure 4) in place of the patient, as it does not tire. In using it, the iris diaphragm should be opened or closed until the pupillary area is the size of a well dilated pupil, or about one-fourth of an inch in diameter.

Fig. 180. Retinoscope

ARRANGEMENT OF THE LIGHT

The light should be arranged either to one side of the patient's head on a level with the ear, or preferably about three inches above the patient's head. The face should always be in a shadow.

POSITION OF OBSERVER

The observer should be stationed one meter in front of the schematic eye or patient (Figure 32) as this is the farthest one can work with convenience. The eye of the observer and that of the patient should be on a level, hence it is convenient to have a screw topped stool for the observer, and a stationary topped one for the patient, a (high chair with back and arms is best for children).

WHAT TO LOOK FOR

Seated one meter in front of the patient, the mirror held in the right or left hand, as is easier for him, and before his corresponding eye, the observer catches the light from the lamp and reflects it back into the patient's eye. The latter should fix a point midway on the observer's brow. If strabismic, the unobserved eye should be covered; otherwise the patient may not maintain fixation.

When the observer catches the emergent or reflected rays on his own retina, he will see a red reflex in the patient's pupil. To get this reflex-it is necessary that the pupil and the sight hole of the mirror coincide, and at first the student may have to close the eye he is not using, but he should learn to keep both eyes open.

After learning to see the retinal reflex the mirror should be tilted on a vertical and horizontal axis. In tilting the mirror on a vertical axis the light reflected on the patient's face will move in the same direction as the mirror is tilted or in the vertical meridian, and in the horizontal meridian when the mirror is tilted on a horizontal axis. *The light on the face always moves in the same direction as the mirror is tilted—i. e. with the mirror.*

The reflex in the pupillary area will move in different directions, presenting different appearances as to form, brilliancy and rapidity of movement in the various refractive conditions of the eye.

From the direction of movement, we learn the following facts, viz: if the reflex moves in the same direction as the mirror or with the light on the face, we have emmetropia, hypermetropia, or myopia of less than one dioptre. If it moves

against the mirror or opposite the light on the
face, we have myopia of more than one dioptre.

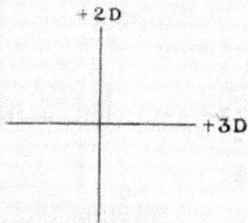

The *more rapid* the
movement of the reflex,
the less the error; and the
slower the movement, the
greater the error.

The *more brilliant* the
reflex, the less the error;
and the dimmer the re-
flex, the greater the error.

Fig. 181. Specimen retinoscopic record cross. (Nu-
gent.)

The *form* or *shape* of
the reflex in simple hypermetropia and myopia
is circular or crescentic in outline, and in the astigmatic errors it is elongated or there is a distinct
band of light across the pupillary area. (See
Pages 198-200.) The long axis of the band is in
the meridian of least error.

The *refracted meridian* is always the one in
which the mirror is moved; and it is best for the
beginner to refract one meridian at a time, as he
will then be less liable to get confused in locating
the meridian of astigmatism if any. In making
his record, it is convenient to make a diagram of
the two principal meridians in the form of a cross,
and to indicate the error found in each meridian.
(Figure 181.)

PRINCIPAL MERIDIANS

The meridians referred to in refraction are
designated on the graduated arc of trial frame
(Figure 50) and correspond to the meridians as

we might imagine them running across the cornea and numbered on its circumference.

While in all circles there are three hundred and sixty degrees (360°) for practical purposes, the trial frame is graduated in divisions of five degrees (5°) beginning always on left side at 0° and running to the right to 180°, one-half only of the circle being graduated. The horizontal meridian is always spoken of as 180°.

When the radii of curvature of the meridians are all equal, the error, if any, is spherical (hypermetropia or myopia). In astigmatism, there is always a meridian of greatest, and one of least curvature of refraction. These meridians are called the principal meridians, and are always 90° apart in regular astigmatism.

By observing the point on the trial frame where the long axis of the band of light strikes, we can judge quite readily the location of the principal meridians, as the long axis of the band lies in the least ametropic meridian and the other is 90° from it.

We often note an oblique movement of the reflex across the pupillary area when we move the mirror vertically or horizontally. The point on the trial frame where the line in which the reflex moves strikes, indicates one of the principal meridians; the other is 90° from it. While this indicates an astigmatic condition, yet we cannot always demonstrate it by retinoscopy, and when an astigmatism is found, cylinders are not always accepted at the trial case.

Again, where they are accepted, it is frequently in the vertical and horizontal meridians. A more accurate way to locate these meridians is to use the axonometer of Thorington. (Figure 182.)

This device is a black disc with a central aperture the size of a dilated pupil and an arrow point on each side of it. It is placed in the trial frame and rotated until the arrow points coincide with the line of movement of the reflex, of the long axis of the band of light,

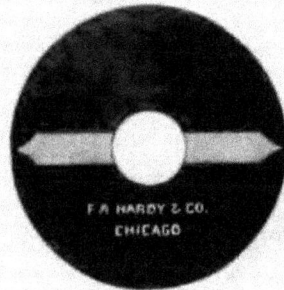

Fig. 182. Axonometer. (Thorington.)

when they will point to one of the principal meridians on the graduated arc, the other meridian being 90 from this.

THE POINT OF REVERSAL

This is the objective point aimed at in retinoscopy. It is the point in front of the eye where emergent rays of light meet or cross, and at this point there will be no movement of the reflex. We establish an artificial point of reversal at which we aim to bring emergent rays of light to a meeting point or focus. This standard point is one meter, and as long as emergent rays do not cross between this point and the patient's eye, the movement of the light reflex is with, and we must place plus lenses in front of the eye until they are brought to a focus at one meter. (See Figs. 183 and 184.)

If on the other hand emergent rays of light cross before they get to our eye, the movement of the reflex will be against, and we must put minus lenses in front of the eye until they are brought to a focus, at one meter. (See Fig. 185.) When this point is found there will be no movement of the light reflex in the pupil. This is the point of reversal, and the lens bringing the rays to a focus at this point represents the refraction of the eye, with — 1 D. added, because of our establishing an artificial myopic far point at 1 meter; or practically, we have rendered the eye 1 D. myopic by working at this distance. If we worked at one-half meter, then we would render the eye 2 D. myopic and would add — 2 D.

After getting the foregoing well fixed in mind, the student should practice observing the reflex and its movement in the schematic eye with the sliding tube in different positions.

APPLICATION OF RETINOSCOPY

For accurate retinoscopy, the accommodation of the patient's eye must be suspended. This means that in cases where asthenopia is marked cyclopegia is necessary. When asthenopia is not marked or where accommodation is naturally suspended simple mydriasis is all that is necessary and this is only for the purpose of getting a large enough pupil so as to get contrasting light and shadow.

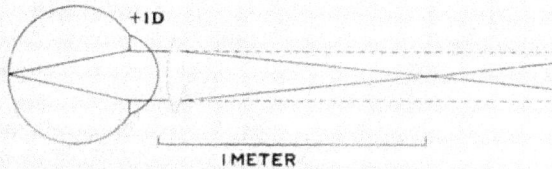

Fig. 183. Emmetropia. (Nugent.)

EMMETROPIA

In this condition we will find the reflex moving with the mirror and plus lenses must be put in front of the eye until there is no movement. A + 1 D. lens will give up a point of no movement, and adding our — 1 D. lens for the one meter distance, we have 0 or emmetropia as the result. (Fig. 183.)

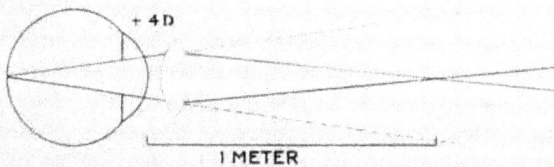

Fig. 184 Hypermetropia. (Nugent.)

HYPERMETROPIA

Here again we will find the reflex moving with the mirror, and plus lenses must be placed in front of the eye to bring the rays of light to a focus at our position of one meter. When we have the plus lens that gives no movement of the reflex, we have established the point of reversal; and if we get the same result in both the vertical and horizontal meridians, we have a simple hypermetropia.

The true amount of error, however, will be represented by the strength of the plus lens found with — 1 D. added, i. e., in a given case it takes a + 4 D. to give the point of reversal in both meridians, adding — 1 D. the result is + 3 D., which will be our starting point at the trial case.

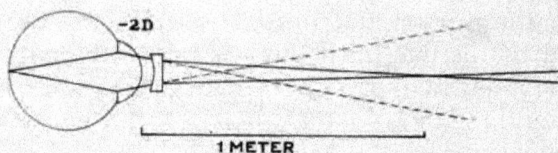

Fig. 185. Myopia. (Nugent.)

MYOPIA

In this we find the reflex moving with the mirror in myopia of less than 1 D. because emergent rays cross beyond one meter, and less than + 1 D. will give us the point of reversal. The addition of — 1 D. then gives less than — 1 D. as the resulting myopia, i. e., + .50 D. gives point of reversal in both meridians, adding — 1 D., the result is — .50 D.

In myopia of more than 1 D. the reflex will always move against the mirror, and we must put — lenses in front of the patient's eye to bring the rays of light to a focus at one meter. The glass which gives no movement of the reflex establishes the point of reversal; and if we get the

same result in both the vertical and horizontal
meridians, we have a simple myopia. (Figure
185.)

The true amount of the error, however, will be
represented by the strength of the — lens with
— 1 D. added, i. e., in a given case it takes a —
3 D. to give the point of reversal in both meridians; adding — 1 D. the result is — 4 D. which
will be our starting point at the trial case.

APPLICATION OF RETINOSCOPY
ASTIGMATISM

In this condition we will find the reflex assuming an elongated or band like appearance reach-
ing across the pupillary area, the long axis of the
elongated reflex or band being in the meridian
of least error and indicating the direction in
which the axis of the correcting cylinder should
be placed.

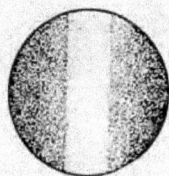

Fig. 186. Retinoscop-
ic illumination and
shadow in Astigma-
tism. (May.)

For practice with the schematic
eye, an astigmatism can be produced showing the band of light
by placing a cylinder in the slot
provided for lenses on the front
end of the model. The student
must remember that when he
uses a plus cylinder he is producing myopic astigmatism, and
when a minus cylinder, hypermetropic astigmatism. Cylinders from .75 D. to 1.50 D. give
best banded reflect when used on a schematic eye.
(Figure 186.)

SIMPLE HYPERMETROPIC ASTIGMATISM

The reflex will move with in both meridians and the banded appearance will be seen early. The meridian in which the long axis lies will be corrected with a + 1 D. lens, indicating emmetropia. The other meridian will be corrected with a stronger + lens and the + lens giving the point for that meridian with — 1 D. added will indicate the amount of astigmatism. (Figure 187.) This result will be the starting point at the trial case, i. e., a + cylinder with the axis in the emmetropic meridian.

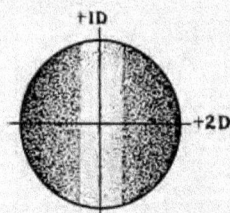

Fig. 187. Simple Hypermetropic Astigmatism. (Nugent.)

+ 1.00 D., in weak meridian + 2.00 D. in strong meridian, adding — 1.00 D. will give 0 in weaker meridian, indicating emmetropia. — 1 D. added to stronger meridian gives + 1.00 D. which requires a + 1.00 D. cylinder axis 90° or in weaker meridian indicated by the band of light.

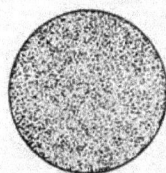

Fig. 188. Compound hypermetropic astigmatism as reflex appears before neutralizing lenses are used. (Nugent.)

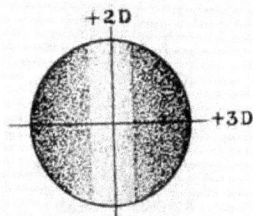

Fig. 189. Compound hypermetropic astigmatism as reflex appears after the weak meridian has been neutralized. (Nugent.)

COMPOUND HYPERMETROPIC ASTIGMATISM (Fig. 188 and 189)

Here the reflex moves in both meridians, but slower in one than in the other. The band of light may not appear until the weaker or faster moving meridian is corrected or nearly so. The result will be a stronger than + 1 D. lens in this meridian, and a stronger one still for the slower moving meridian, i. e., weak meridian + 2 D. strong meridian + 3 D. adding — 1 D. will give a + 1 D. for the weaker and a + 1 D. sphere with a + 1 D. cylinder with its axis in the weaker meridian or + 1.00 + 1.00 ax 90°. (See Nugent's Rule.)

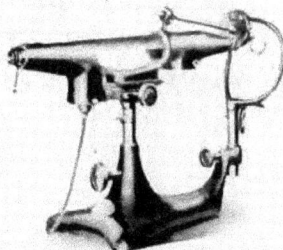

Fig. 189a. Geneva Ophthalmoscope and Retinoscope (descriptive pamphlet accompanies the instrument).

+1.00

-.50

+1.00

+1.50

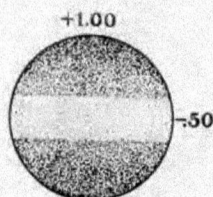

Fig. 190. Simple Myopic Astigmatism of more than 1 D. (Nugent.)

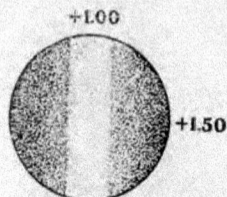

Fig. 191. Simple Hypermetropic
Astigmatism of less than 1 D.
(Nugent.)

SIMPLE MYOPIC ASTIGMATISM

If the astigmatism is more than 1 D. we will
find the reflex moving with the mirror in one
meridian and a + 1 D. lens will give the point
or reversal: adding — 1 D. gives emmetropia
for that meridian. The opposite meridian, however, will give an against the mirror movement
of the reflex and it will take a minus lens to give
the point of reversal, and adding a — 1 D. will
give one more dioptre of myopia for that meridian. This lens, a cylinder with the axis in the
emmetropic meridian, will be our starting point
at the trial case. If the myopic meridian is less
than 1 D. the motion of the reflex will be with
the mirror: the point of reversal will be indicated
by a + lens of less than 1 D. and the result will
be estimated the same as in myopia, but in one
meridian at a time. (Figure 191.)

COMPOUND MYOPIC ASTIGMATISM

If the myopia is more than 1.00 D. the reflex
will move against the mirror in both meridians,
but at different rates. The more rapidly moving

−2D

−1D

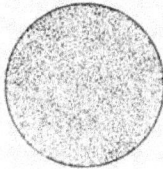

Fig. 192. Compound myopic astigmatism showing appearance of reflex before neutralizing lens is used.
(Nugent.)

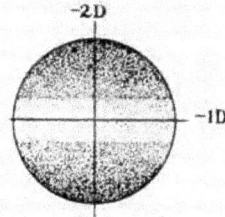

Fig. 193. Compound myopic astigmatism showing appearance of band
of light after meridian of least
error has been neutralized. 2 D
Sph. 1 D cyl. × 180. See Nugent's Rule. Page 202.

reflex will be in the meridian of least error and the
more slowly moving reflex will be in the one of
greatest error. Estimating each meridian separately, and adding — 1 D. for our distance of 1
meter, as in all other cases, we have as a result a
minus sphere combined with a minus cylinder
with its axis in the weaker meridian. Figures
192 and 193.

MIXED ASTIGMATISM

In this condition we will find the two meridians
indicating different denominations of refraction.
—i. e. myopia in one and hyperopia in the other.
Each meridian should be estimated separately
and — 1 D. be added to the correction found
for each meridian. Figs. 184 and 185. The correcting lens obtained by combining the two lenses
into one is called a crossed cylinder, and the axes
of these cylinders are 90 apart or at right angles.
Crossed cylinder, however, is not often used, the
correction being made by a combination of a
sphere and cylinder. See Nugent's Rule.

IRREGULAR ASTIGMATISM

Retinoscopy does not give very satisfactory results in this condition. It is usually caused by opacities on the cornea or lens, and these so scatter the rays of light that no distinct direction of movement can be made out. However, by persistence a result may be obtained which is useful as a foundation in getting a manifest correction that will be beneficial to the patient.

LENSES USED

In estimating the refraction by retinoscopy the lenses actually necessary are spheres only, as we estimate first one meridian, then the other. Some refractionists, however, prefer to use cylinders in the estimation of astigmatism. This is unnecessary and is apt to be confusing because of the many surfaces for reflections of light.

NUGENT'S RULE: The following rule devised by Dr. O. B. Nugent for the purpose of writing formulae from net retinoscopic findings, is concise, accurate, easy to understand and memorize, and is applicable to each and all of the results obtained by the retinoscope.

THE RULE: Choose the numeral from one (lesser) meridian for the sphere. Now subtract this number from the numeral in the other (greater) meridian. The remainder is the strength and sign of the cylinder, the axis of which is indicated by the meridian from which sph. was chosen. (Figure 194.)

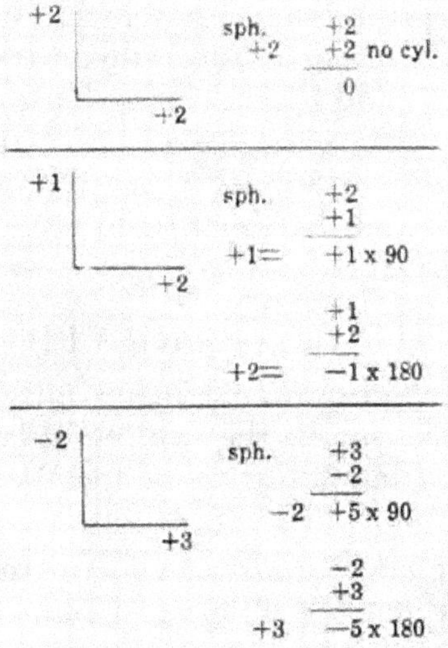

```
+2 |
   |              sph.   +2
   |               +2    +2   no cyl.
   |              _____
   |_____                0
       +2


+1 |
   |              sph.   +2
   |                     +1
   |                    _____
   |                +1=  +1 x 90
   |_____
       +2
                         +1
                         +2
                        _____
                    +2=  −1 x 180


−2 |
   |              sph.   +3
   |                     −2
   |                    _____
   |                −2   +5 x 90
   |_____
       +3
                         −2
                         +3
                        _____
                    +3   −5 x 180
```

Fig. 194. Nugent's Rule

PRACTICAL WAY OF FINDING THE POINT OF REVERSAL

It has been found that, as the point of no movement of the reflex is hard to recognize and is generally ambiguous, the most practical way of finding the point of reversal is to take the half-way point between the strongest lens with which the reflex distinctly moves in the same direction and the weakest lens with which it distinctly moves in the opposite direction. i. e. in a given case the reflex moves without a lens, and the strongest lens with which it moves distinctly with is a + 4 D., the weakest with which it moves distinctly against is a + 4.50 D., or the half-way point between the two is + 4.25 D., or the point of reversal. Again, if the reflex without lenses moves against, and the strongest lense with which it moves against is a — 5 D., and the weakest with which it moves with is a — 5.50 D., then the half-way point between them is — 5.25 D. or the point of reversal.

SPHERIC ABERRATION

This is a condition that often puzzles the beginner. Because of the widely dilated pupil, there are two distinct areas of light and shadow, a peripheral one and a central one.

In positive aberration the central reflex moves with, and the peripheral area of light or shadow, against the mirror.

In negative aberration, (conic cornea) the central reflex moves against and the peripheral one with the mirror.

If the student will get in the habit of always observing the movement of the reflex throughout a four to five millimeter area at the apex of the cornea he will not be bothered by these conditions. We do not care for the refraction in the periphery as this area is covered by the iris, hence, we disregard it.

Spheric aberration is frequently annoying in estimating astigmatism in the vertical meridian. As in astigmatism the reflex is banded, we find in this condition a band of light running horizontally across the pupil, with the ends of the ring obliterated by the iris. This gives us the appear-

ance of three bands; and when the eye is tilted
slightly up or down, one of the bands is not seen,
and we find only two bands which come together
and separate like the blades of a pair of scissors
as we tilt the mirror vertically. The condition
is called the scissors movement, and is sometimes
ascribed as being due to a tilting of the lens in
its fossa. This gives another reason why we
should stick to the central reflex. The lens used
to correct this error with the retinoscope is one
that will keep the two "bands of light" together,
or nearly so.

VALUE OF RETINOSCOPY

The value of retinoscopy is in the fact that it
is a method by which we get the refraction of
the eye objectively. This makes it indispensable
in young (Hypermetropic) children, with strabismus or other condition where glasses are necessary, and illiterates from any cause, who cannot
tell us what lenses they see best with at the trial
case.

MYDRIATICS AND CYCLOPEGICS

For many cases of refraction, the use of drugs
is necessary for dilating the pupil and suspending
the accommodation and we should have a clear
idea in our minds as to what we can expect from
those drugs and how to use them.

A mydriatic is a drug which dilates the pupil.

A cyclopegic not only dilates the pupil but
paralyzes the ciliary muscle.

All cyclopegics are mydriatics, but all mydriatics are not cyclopegics.

The following table gives the different mydriatics and cyclopegics with duration of the paralysis:

Euphthalmin—purely mydriatic.

Cocoain—purely mydriatic. Occasionally slightly cyclopegic.

Homatropin—complete paralysis—2 hours; complete recovery 2 days.

Scopolamin—complete paralysis—½ hour; complete recovery 4 days.

Hyoscyamin—complete paralysis. 3 days; complete recovery 8 days.

Duboisin—complete paralysis, 2 days; complete recovery 8 days.

Atropin—complete paralysis, 2 days; complete recovery 15 days.

Solution of proper strength of those drugs when dropped into the eye, in a short time begins to give effect, by acting on the nerve endings of the sphincter muscles of the iris and ciliary body, paralyzing their action, thus producing dilated pupil and suspension of accommodation.

Atropin, is the most reliable cyclopegic, and where accurate suspension of accommodation is desired should be used. It is used in solutions varying from two to ten grains to the ounce. The two grains solution for children up to the age of ten years and the four grains solution from this age upward. The stronger solution is generally used only where the weaker solution has failed to give complete cyclopegia.

There is very little danger of getting toxic effects from the drug, if care is used in closing the puncta by pressure over the inner canthi with the thumb and finger deeply enough to close the canaliculi and instilling the solution (not dropping it) into the eye at the external canthi. In this way the solution is kept from getting into the throat, through the nasal ducts, swallowed, and taken up by the stomach. The symptoms of poisoning are dry throat, flushed face, and rapid pulse, and when they occur the drug should be discontinued.

The action of this drug while profound is slow, and it should be dropped into the eyes three or four times a day for three days, when the cyclopegia is usually complete, and the patient ready for refraction. If the cyclopegia is not complete, it can be used for a day or two longer. In fact, when the patient is using atropine, we might as well use it long enough to get two examinations approximating each other pretty closely, when we can feel certain we have obtained the best result.

Homatropin, is the most transient cyclopegic we have and is very useful in the examination of adults, (and even good results can be secured in children) where time cannot be given to the use of atropin. For use in the office we are accustomed to use the No. 342 gelatin disc of Wyeth.

It is used also in 2 per-cent solution in water or oil (castor or olive) one drop being instilled into the conjunctival sac every five minutes six to eight times when, after twenty to thirty minutes, the action is supposed to be complete and the patient ready for refraction.

The practical way to use the discs is to pick up one with a pledget of cotton, wound on a toothpick or probe and dampened with boric acid solution or sterile water, and place it in the lower conjunctival sac. If the cotton is quite wet the disc will readily adhere to the conjunctiva. Let the patient keep his eyes closed for half an hour (best by bandaging), use a separate disc in each eye, and keep the eyes closed again; action will be obtained in one hour from the time first disc is used. Some prefer to use a disc every twenty minutes for three times, waiting twenty minutes after the last one when the patient is ready for refraction.

Scopolamin is quite a favorite with some oculists, but its action in our experience is no better than homatropin and the effect is more prolonged. It is advised to use it in a one grain to the ounce solution, one drop of which solution instilled into the conjunctival sac is supposed to give complete cyclopegia in one-half hour.

Hyoscyamin is not often used.

Duboisin is useful more as a substitute for atropin, when there seems to be an idiosyncrasy for the latter drug. This is manifested by a marked conjunctival irritation with erythema. Duboisin is best used in a 1 per cent ointment.

CHAPTER XII

MEASUREMENT OF LENSES, PRE-SCRIPTION WRITING, TRANSPO-SITION AND FRAME FITTING

The determination of the proper correction is not nearly all that is necessary in the treatment of refractive errors; but, if success in this important branch of therapeutics is to be attained, as much care must be taken in selecting the form of lens suited to the case and in properly mounting it before the eye as is used in doing the refraction.

FORMS OF LENSES: In the early days of the specialty, spherical lenses were either biconvex or biconcave as the case might be, as shown in Figures 195 and 196.

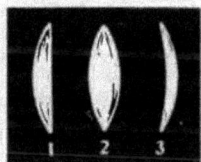

Fig. 195. Convex Lenses. 1, Plano-Convex; 2, Bi-Convex; 3, Convex Meniscus. (May.)

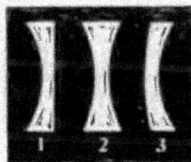

Fig. 196. Concave Lenses. 1, Plano-Concave; 2, Bi-Concave; 3, Concave Meniscus. (May.)

For cosmetic reasons and for the purpose of bringing the periphery of the lens nearer the eye the plano convex and concave. (Figures 195 and 196) were devised. The meniscus form, even with only the usual plus or minus one and twenty-five hundreths D. base surface has been found so much more satisfactory than the earlier forms that of recent years much deeper meniscus forms, six dioptre base surface or even in some cases nine dioptre base surface have come into general use.

This form has been found to be comparatively free from annoying reflections, to bring the edge of the lens quite near the eye and to have the added advantage of causing the eye to look more nearly at right angles to its surface.

TORIC LENS: The deep meniscus lens has proven so satisfactory that there has been developed a demand for a similar lens in cylindrical correction which has been met by the toric lens.

By varying the radii of curvature any desired difference of refractive power between the two meridians, the cylindrical correction may be produced. Then by grinding a neutralizing sphere on the original plane surface, the spherical correction will result.

EXAMPLE: If it is desired to make a + 1 D. sph. ⌒ + 1 cyl. ax 90 in the toric form, a blank is selected in which the meridian of least curvature, called the case curve, has a refractive power of 6 D and the stronger one has the refractive power of + 7 D. Remembering that the dioptric power of a lens is equal to the algebraic sum of the two surfaces expressed dioptrically, we now grind a minus 50 sphere on the plane surface producing the desired strength, and cut the lens from the blank with its weakest meridian at 90°.

Theoretically, a toric lens need not be of the deep meniscus form, but practically they always are so, because the sole purpose for which they are made is to obtain the advantages resulting from the meniscus form.

TRANSPOSITION OF LENSES: While in practice, when prescribing toric lenses, it is safer for the oculist to leave the above calculations to the optician; it is necessary that he have a thorough knowledge of transposition, the combining of two lenses into one or of changing the form of a lens to a more desirable one while retaining the same dioptric power.

RULES FOR TRANSPOSING: Rule 1. To combine plus spheres and cylinders or minus spheres and cylinders to produce a periscopic lens, take the sum of the sphere and cylinder for the new sphere and retain the cylinder with its sign changed and axis moved 90 degrees.

EXAMPLES: 1. $+ 1 \supset + 1$ cyl. ax. 105 $= + 2$
   sph. $\supset - 1$ ax. 15.

   2. $- 2$ sph. $\supset - 50$ cyl. ax. 180 $=$
   $- 2.50$ sph. $\supset + 50$ cyl. ax. 90.

Rule 2. To combine spheres and cylinders of opposite signs, take their numerical difference for the new sphere giving it the sign of the stronger original lens and retain the cylinder changing its sign and moving its axis 90 degrees.

EXAMPLES: 1. $+ 3$ sph. $\supset - 2$ cyl. ax. 90 $=$
   $+ 1$ sph. $\supset + 2$ cyl. ax. 180;

   2. $+ .50$ sph. $\supset - 2.50$ cyl. ax. 150
   $= - 2$ sph. $\supset + 2.50$ cyl. ax. 60;

3. — 3 sph. ⊃ + 3 cyl. ax. 100 =
+ 2.00 sph. ⊃ — 1 cyl. ax. 10;
4. — 1 sph. ⊃ + 3 cyl. ax. 100 =
+ 2.00 sph. ⊃ — 3 cyl. ax. 10.

Rule 3. To convert cylinders, either plus or minus, to sphere cylinders, use sphere of same power and sign and retain cylinder with sign changed and axis moved 90 degrees.

EXAMPLES: 1. + 2.25 cyl. ax. 90 ⊃ + 2.25 sph.
= — 2.25 cyl. ax. 180.
2. — 1.75 cyl. ax. 180 ⊃ — 1.75 sph.
= + 1.75 cyl. ax. 90.

Rule 4. To change crossed cylinders of like sign to sphere cylinders, take the weaker cylinder for the sphere retaining its sign and the difference between the original cylinders for the new numerical cylinders retaining the sign and axis of the stronger.

EXAMPLES: 1. + 1 cyl. ax. 100 ⊃ + 2 cyl. ax. 10
= + 1 sph. ⊃ + 1 cyl. ax. 10:
2. — 2 cyl. ax. 170 ⊃ — 1 cyl. ax. 80
= — 1 sph. ⊃ — 1 cyl. ax. 170.

or, take stronger cylinder for sphere retaining its sign and the numerical difference between the original cylinders for the new cylinder, changing the sign and giving it the axis of the stronger one.

EXAMPLES: 1. + 2.00 cyl. ax. 180 ⊃ + 3 cyl.
ax. 90 = + 3.00 sph. ⊃ — 1 cyl.
ax. 180;
2. — 3.00 cyl. ax. 180 ⊃ — 2 cyl.
ax. 90 = — 3.00 sph. ⊃ + 1 cyl.
ax. 180.

Rule 5. To change crossed cylinders of unlike

sign to sphere-cylinders: Take either cylinder for
the sphere retaining its sign and the algebraic
sum of both cylinders for the new cylinder giving
it the sign and axis of the cylinder not used for
the sphere.

EXAMPLES: 1. $+$ 2 cyl. ax. 90 $\bigcirc$ — 1 cyl. ax. 180
$=$ $+$ 2.00 sph. $\bigcirc$ — 3 cyl. ax.
180.

2. or — 1 sph. $\bigcirc$ $+$ 3.00 cyl. ax. 90.

MEASUREMENT OF PATIENT'S GLASSES: While
it is perhaps unwise for a beginner to risk the
possibility of biasing his judgment by measuring
the glasses the patient has been wearing before
completing his own examination, no examination
is to be regarded as
complete that does
not c o n t a i n a
record of the pre-
s c r i p t i o n he is
wearing.

To d e t e r-
mine the strength
of a spectacle lens,
one may use the
general lens meas-
ure (Brayton pa-
tent Figure 197).

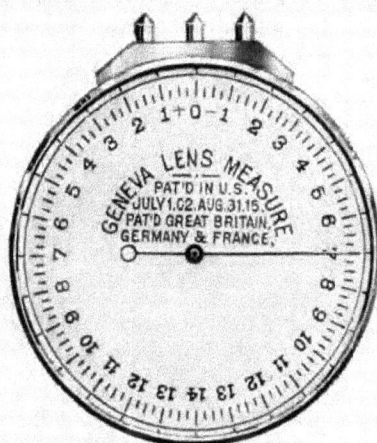

Fig. 197. Lens Measure

which gives the curvature of the two surfaces
instantly so that the dioptric strength may be
found by a simple calculation, or their strength
may be determined by neutralization which process all operators should understand.

NEUTRALIZATION OF LENSES: In neutralizing a lens, the first step is to determine whether it is convex or concave and whether or not it contains a cylinder in which event its axis must be located and the test for plus and minus made in and at right angles to this meridian.

To determine whether the lens is convex or concave, if its curvature is not so great as to make its character obvious, look through it at a distant object which will be observed to seem to move as the lens is moved slightly from side to side. If the object moves opposite the direction of lens movement, it is convex; and if in the same direction, it is concave. Should there be no movement, it must be a plano.

To determine the presence or absence of a cylinder, look through the lens at some object, preferably a line that cannot be seen in its entirety while looking through the lens, meanwhile, slowly rotating it. If the line remains continuous the lens contains no cylinder; but if the line becomes broken during the rotation, a cylinder is present and its axis lies in one of the two meridians in which the line was not broken.

With the character of the lens determined, it is neutralized by placing spheres of the opposite sign in contact with it and repeating the movement test, varying strength of neutralization lens until there is noted and recorded that having the strength of the lens under examination, using, of course, the opposite sign. When a cylinder is present the same procedure is followed save that it must be done in both principal meridians obtaining a result in crossed cylinders which may be transposed according to the rules just given.

FRAME FITTING: *Extreme importance*

With the best possible form of lenses selected, they must be mounted accurately, safely and attractively before the patient's eyes. The choice between the eye glasses and spectacles, either of which may be rimless or in frames, may usually be left to the patient with certain reservations, save in the case of young children who invariably should be given frame spectacles.

CHOICE OF MOUNTING: If the patient have no astigmatism and so desires he may be given regular eye glasses; but if he has an astigmatism it is safer for him to wear either a finger piece mounting or spectacles, since the regular eye glasses get out of adjustment readily and the cylinders off axis.

Having determined on the form in which the lenses are to be mounted, the next step is to select the size of mounting best suited to the patient's needs. This can best be done by means of fitting sets of standard sizes of bridges which can be procured in either eye glasses, (Figure 198) or spectacles (Figure 199) from any wholesale optician.

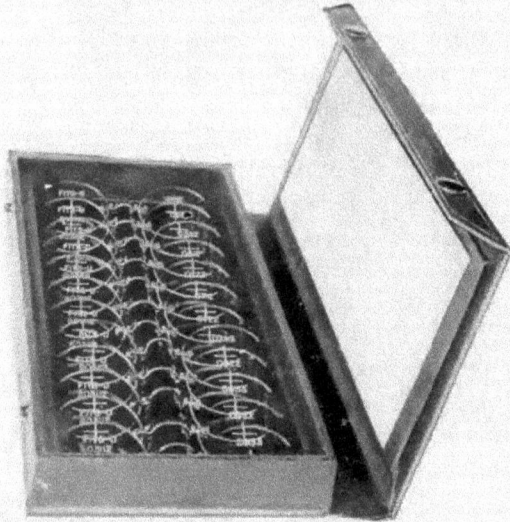

Fig. 198. Nose Mountings

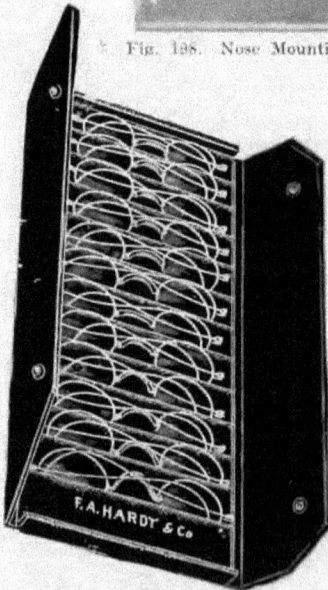

Fig. 199. Spectacle Frames

INTERPUPIL-
LARY DISTANCE:
We now deter-
mine the inter-
pupillary distance
by actual meas-
urement, usually
measuring from
the inner margin
of one pupil to
to the outer mar-
gin of the other
with the patient
looking at the dis-
tance at which
the glasses are to
be used.

In practice the patient looks over the operator's head for distance and at his nose for near. When measuring the inter-pupillary distance one should remember too, that the eyes are not always equidistant from the mid line, and, if so, order his mounting of frame accordingly.

SELECTION OF LENSES: With the individual mounting selected and the inter-pupillary distance known, we select a lens of such size and shape (illustration of which may be found in any optical catalogue) as will place their optical centers exactly before the pupils and at the same time look well on the patient's face. If there be a great disparity between the inter-pupillary distance and the size of the face and features, or one eye be farther from the mid-line than the other, decentering of one or both lenses may be necessary.

MEASUREMENT FOR SPECTACLES: When ordering spectacles, in addition to the inter-pupillary distance, one must determine the distance between temples, also the temple length.

FRAME FITTING IN PRESBYOPIA: Originally ametropic presbyopic patients were given two pair of glasses; but at present, whenever possible, the distant and near correction are placed in the same mounting in some form of bifocal. Emmetropic presbyopes also frequently object to the blurred distant vision when they look up from near work and avoid it by adding their presbyopia correction to a plano for distance. Several forms of bifocals have been devised, the efforts for improvements being directed to making the junction of the near and distant corection invisible: but the one point that must be remembered is, with the main portion of the correcting lens centered for distance, to have the reading scales decentered inward two millimeters.

ADJUSTMENTS: With the greatest possible care in frame fitting adjustments will be found necessary and one will need to provide himself with suitable pliers and learn to use them. A few dollars invested in a supply of the various mountings and spectacles in the cheaper grades and time spent in adjusting them to different faces will well repay one in the satisfaction to his patients that the wearing of a proper correction properly mounted always brings.

INDEX

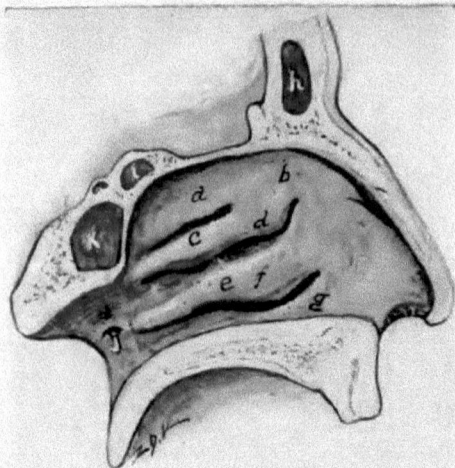

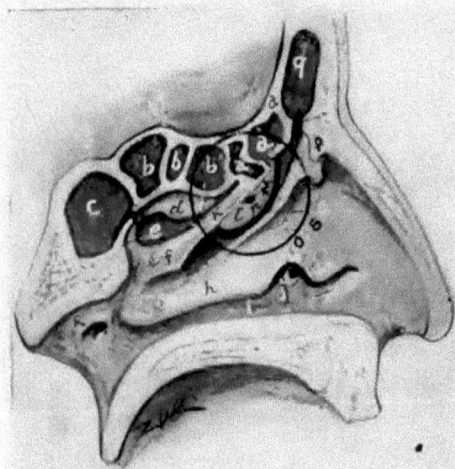

www.ingramcontent.com/pod-product-compliance
Lightning Source LLC
Chambersburg PA
CBHW060547200326
41521CB00007B/514